ESSENTI OLOGY

£14·95

ESSENTIALS OF MEDICAL MYCOLOGY

E. Glyn V. Evans
BSc, PhD, MI Biol
Senior Lecturer in Medical Mycology,
University of Leeds and General Infirmary at Leeds, UK

James C. Gentles
BSc, PhD, FRSE
Emeritus Professor of Medical Mycology,
University of Glasgow, UK

Churchill Livingstone
EDINBURGH LONDON MELBOURNE AND NEW YORK 1985

CHURCHILL LIVINGSTONE
Medical Division of Longman Group Limited

Distributed in the United States of America by Churchill Livingstone Inc., 1560 Broadway, New York, N.Y. 10036, and by associated companies, branches and representatives throughout the world.

First published 1985

ISBN 0 443 02505 3

British Library Cataloguing in Publication Data
Evans, E. Glyn V.
Essentials of medical mycology. — (Churchill Livingstone medical text)
1. Mycoses
I. Title II. Gentles, James C.
616.9'69 RC117

Library of Congress Cataloging in Publication Data
Evans, E. Glyn V.
Essentials of medical mycology.
Bibliography: p.
Includes index.
1. Mycoses. 2. Medical mycology. I. Gentles, James C. II. Title.
RC117.E93 1985 616.9'69 84–23143

Produced by Longman Singapore Publishers (Pte) Ltd.
Printed in Singapore.

PREFACE

During the last few decades it has become increasingly clear that diseases of fungal origin are of major importance. Superficial mycoses are widespread and have increased in incidence since the introduction of occlusive synthetic materials for clothing and footwear and the greater availability and frequency of use of communal bathing facilities. There has also been a dramatic increase in iatrogenic and potentially fatal opportunistic mycoses in debilitated patients treated with, for example, cytotoxic and immunosuppressive drugs, corticosteroids or broad-spectrum antibiotics, which are now also commonly used in conjunction with specialized techniques such as cardiac and transplant surgery. Furthermore, because of the speed and ease of intercontinental travel and its use by large numbers of individuals, certain mycotic diseases now occur relatively frequently in places far removed from their endemic regions. There is a need, therefore, for students and laboratory workers in medicine and microbiology to have a greater awareness and understanding of the fungal diseases of man than is provided during their formal courses of instruction or training. A number of textbooks which cover the subject in depth are available but a relatively inexpensive text providing basic information on the characteristics, distribution, diagnosis and treatment of the mycoses and suitable for use by those for whom medical mycology is a fringe interest has not been produced. It is hoped that this book despite its brevity and unavoidable generalizations will fill this gap and help to stimulate a much needed interest in the subject.

1985

E.G.V.E
J.C.G.

ACKNOWLEDGEMENTS

We are most grateful to the staffs of the departments of medical mycology in Leeds and Glasgow for their continued support and in particular to Mr R.A. Forster for helpful discussion and assistance with the illustrations, to Mr A.P. West for production of line drawings, to Mr I. McKie for photographic assistance and to Mr A.M. Sharp for help with the indexing. We wish also to express our thanks and appreciation to Mrs Dorothy Newton for her considerable patience during the production of the typed manuscript.

CONTENTS

NOMENCLATURE OF THE MYCOSES

There are no rules or regulations governing the nomenclature of the mycoses and most disease names have been formed by adding the suffix -osis or -mycosis to the generic name of the causal fungus. This system is not entirely satisfactory because the same fungus may cause a number of different diseases whilst the same disease may be caused by a number of different fungi and furthermore the names of fungi are subject to change. Within recent years efforts have been made by the Medical Research Council* in Britain, the International Society for Human and Animal Mycology† and the World Health Organization‡ to produce lists of internationally acceptable names and there has been a considerable measure of agreement between these authorities, at least for the most important diseases. These recommendations have been followed in the preparation of this text and where there is disagreement our choice of name has been made on the basis of personal choice or common usage in Great Britain. In such cases the synonyms are also given.

* Medical Research Council 1977 Nomenclature of fungi pathogenic to man and animals. MRC Memorandum no. 23, 4th edn. Her Majesty's Stationary Office, London

† International Society for Human and Animal Mycology 1980 Nomenclature of mycoses. Sabouraudia 18: 78–84

‡ Council for International Organizations of Medical Sciences 1982 Infectious diseases. Part 2 Mycoses. In: International nomenclature of diseases, vol 11

Chapter One
THE NATURE OF FUNGI

Fungi constitute a large group of eukaryotic organisms which depend for their nutrients on previously elaborated organic materials on which they live as saprophytes or parasites. They show considerable diversity in size and morphology but no matter how large or small a fungal mass may be, it is never vascularized and is composed of cellular elements of the same basic form. These cells consist of a firm, mainly polysaccharide wall with an inner cell membrane surrounding cytoplasm which encloses the nuclei (usually two or more), food reserves (fat, oil or glycogen) and vacuoles filled with cell sap. Such basic cell-units may exist separately as yeasts but they are more often joined together to form filaments (hyphae) as in moulds; in certain instances the hyphae may become closely associated to form a pseudo-tissue, such as in toadstools and mushrooms. Such gross differences in form have led to the popular classification of fungi into yeasts, moulds and toadstools but, in effect, these do not differ fundamentally one from the other. Under certain conditions yeasts may become filamentous and conversely moulds may grow and multiply as yeasts whilst toadstools and mushrooms grow as widely separate filaments for much of the time, producing conspicuous fruiting bodies only after a considerable period of consolidation on the substrate.

The mycological classification of fungi is based primarily on the method of sexual reproduction. However, one group is an artificial one and contains all the fungi for which no method of sexual reproduction has been discovered either because of incomplete or unsatisfactory methods of study or because the fungus has become adapted to exist without recourse to a sexual state.

As well as the sexual reproductive bodies which are usually conspicuous in nature, fungi form many other distinctive structures. Some are purely vegetative and formed by the modification of single cells or aggregated masses of cells but the most common structures formed are asexual spores which are usually produced in large numbers.

The sequence of events in the development of a fungus consists of colonization of the substrate by vegetative growth followed by the production of units, usually asexual spores, for rapid dispersal to other substrates. The fungus then prepares to undergo the period of rest which will become necessary either because of depletion of nutrients or the onset of other adverse conditions and it does so by reproducing sexually, or by forming resistant vegetative structures, or both.

VEGETATIVE STRUCTURES

The individual filaments of a fungus are termed hyphae and the interwoven mass of vegetative hyphae is known as mycelium. Growth takes place at the hyphal tips which are densely filled with cytoplasm and contain a large number of nuclei. A regular system of lateral branching, manifest as the hyphae mature, is also initiated at the hyphal tips where the cell wall is thin and plastic. As the hyphae mature, cross-walls or septa are formed and the cells become vacuolated with the cytoplasm reduced to a thin layer containing one or more nuclei. The cross-walls of septate hyphae usually have a central pore which allows free movement of contents including nuclei. In one large group of fungi the hyphae characteristically remain aseptate existing as a single multinucleate cell or coenocyte (Fig. 1.1a–c).

Yeasts are predominantly unicellular and uninucleate with round, oval or elongate cells. A few species reproduce by fission but most yeasts propagate by a process of budding with a daughter cell or

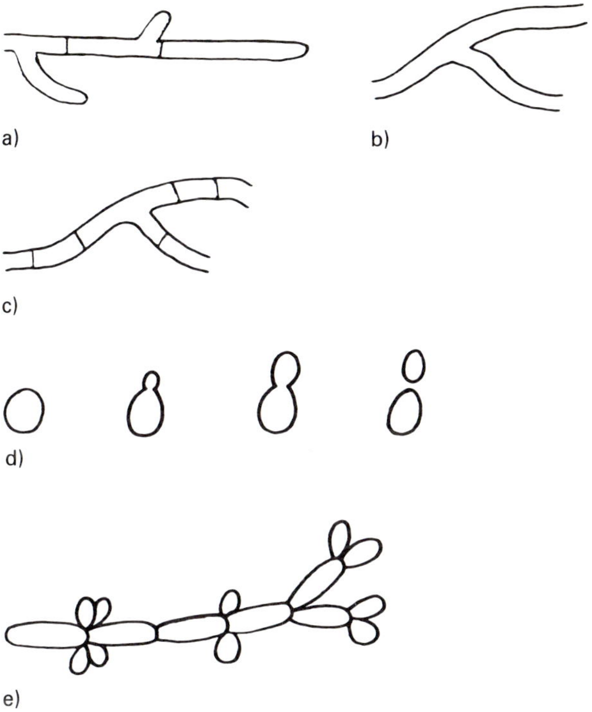

Fig. 1.1 Diagrammatic representation of vegetative forms of fungi: (a) hyphal tip with lateral branching; (b) aseptate (coenocytic) hypha; (c) septate hypha; (d) yeast cells showing stages in budding; (e) yeast pseudomycelium (pseudohypha)

blastospore arising on the surface of the parent. Usually the daughter cells separate from the parent but under certain conditions they may elongate and remain attached to form a chain of cells or pseudomycelium. True mycelium may also be formed by a number of yeast species (Fig. 1.1d, e).

In mycelial fungi, individual cells, or similar units cut off in coenocytic hyphae, may become enriched with nutritive materials, form a thick resistant wall and enter a period of rest; these are chlamydospores. They are usually larger than vegetative cells, and may be formed singly or in groups in an intercalary or a terminal position. Another unicellular vegetative spore is the arthrospore formed by the production of numerous cross-septa to give chains of small cuboidal spores with slightly thickened walls which disarticulate when mature. Chlamydospores and arthrospores (Fig. 1.2) since they are produced directly by sep-

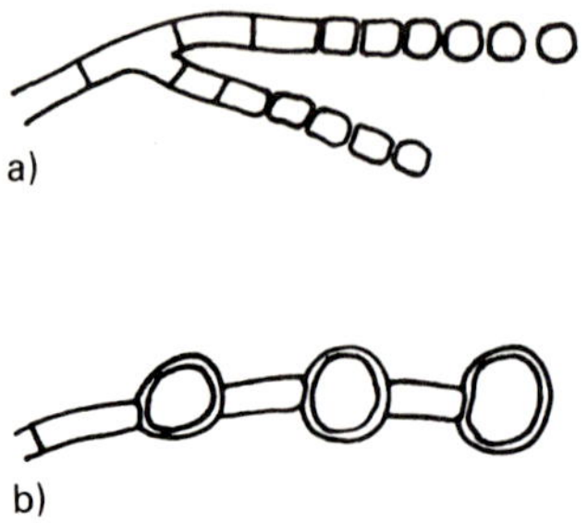

Fig. 1.2 Vegetative spores (thallospores) of fungi: (a) arthrospores; (b) chlamydospores

tation of a hypha may also be referred to as thallospores. Other structures are formed by modification of the hyphae rather than the individual cell. A sclerotium develops from a mass of hyphae which have become aggregated to form a tissue, with cells variously thickened and modified so as to lose their filamentous character. The outermost cells are usually much thickened and resistant. Groups of hyphae may also associate closely to form rhizomorphs, which are branched, rope-like structures which enable the fungus to spread over a considerable distance from one source of nutrient to another. In this case the hyphae lie parallel to one another and do not lose their individual characteristics, but again the outermost hyphae are much thickened and resistant.

ASEXUAL REPRODUCTION

Asexual spores are usually produced in great numbers following rapid and frequent mitotic nuclear division. They may be borne within an envelope or sporangium in which case they are sporangiospores or they may be borne exogenously when they are called conidiospores or simply conidia (Fig. 1.3). As distinct from vegetative spores they are usually formed on specialized structures called sporophores which differ from the vegetative hyphae in one or more characters such as limited growth, vertical position, nature of cell wall, shape of cells or characteristic branching. They may arise singly or be aggregated together to form compound sporophores such as the coremium in which individual spore-bearing hyphae are bound closely together with the fertile spore-bearing parts free at the tip. A number of fungi protect the sporophores by enclosing them in a pycnidium, a globose or flask-shaped structure with a pseudo-parenchymatous wall and an opening or ostiole through which the asexual conidia (pycnidiospores) are released.

SEXUAL REPRODUCTION

The sexual or perfect state of a fungus involves the fusion of cells (plasmogamy) followed by the fusion of two nuclei (karyogamy) and a subsequent meiosis or reduction division. In contrast to animals and higher plants, fungi are haploid and meiosis therefore takes place following fusion and not prior to the production of the sex cells or gametes. Except in certain yeasts, the diploid state is relatively short-lived.

The way in which the nuclei are brought together, the subsequent development of the zygote and the type of sexual spore produced varies considerably among the different groups of fungi. The fusion may occur between motile gametes or undifferentiated hyphae or between specialized gametangia which may be morphologically distinguishable as male and female organs. In lower fungi the nuclei usually fuse within the cell in which they are brought together but in more advanced fungi the fusion of nuclei is delayed. Both the nuclei and the cells that contain them undergo a period of multiplication which gives rise to a phase of binucleate (dikaryotic) cells before fusion of the nuclear pairs (dikaryons) eventually takes place.

Within all classes of fungi there are some species in which a single spore may produce a thallus (vegetative body) which is capable of reproducing sexually. Such fungi are homothallic. In others the sexual state can be formed only when union occurs between the cells or gametes of compatible pairs of thalli which have arisen from separate spores. These are heterothallic species. As the thalli of heterothallic species are usually morphologically alike and can be identified only by their mating characteristics they are usually designated '+' and '−' strains. Sexual spores are usually resistant structures and in the

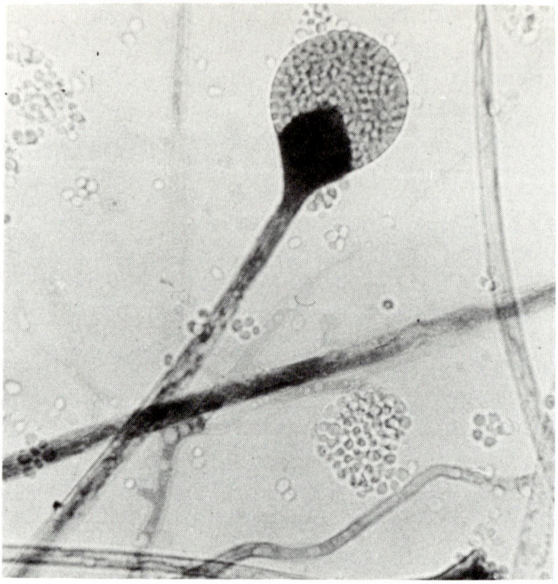

a)

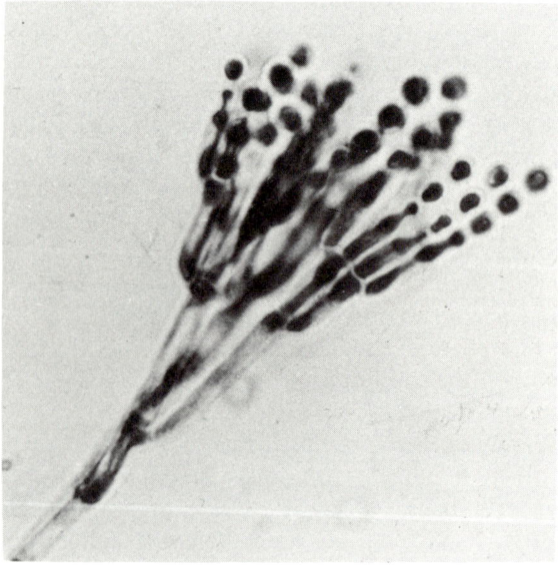

b)

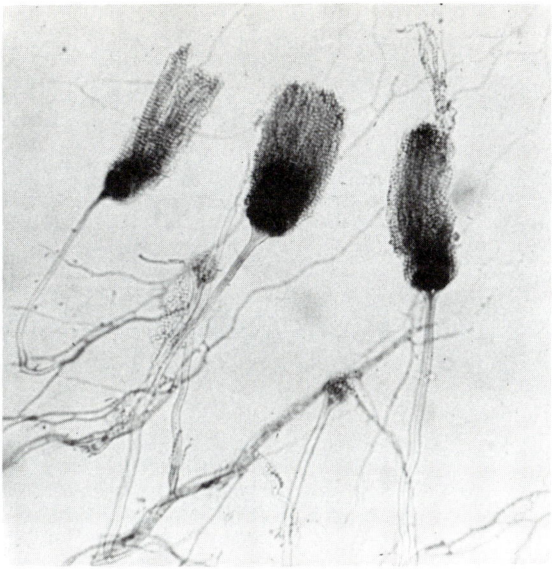

c)

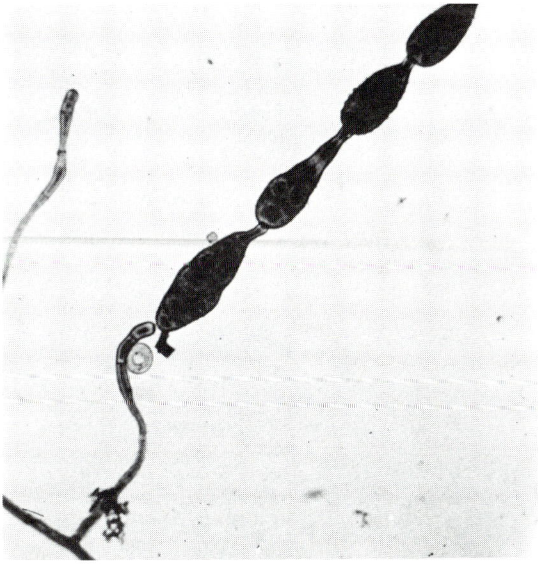

d)

Fig. 1.3 Asexual reproductive forms of fungi: (a) Sporangium of *Mucor* (× 320) (b) Asymmetrically branched sporophore (conidiophore) of *Penicillium* (× 480) (c) Conidiophores of *Aspergillus* with swollen tips and chains of conidia (× 50) (d) Simple conidiophore and chain of mutlicelled conidia of *Alternaria* (× 240) (Cotton Blue/Lactophenol) more advanced fungi they are frequently protected within fruiting bodies which vary in size, shape and complexity. The major characteristics of the various groups of fungi are given in Table 1.1.

Table 1.1 Outline classification of fungi and major characteristics of the groups (after Ainsworth 1973)†

	Sub-divisions	
Lower Fungi (Phycomycetes)	Mastigomycotina	Mycelium, if formed, coenocytic. Asexual spores formed in sporangium. Spores and/or gametes motile. Sexual spores varied in form.
	Zygomycotina	Mycelium coenocytic. Asexual spores in sporangia. Spores non-motile. Sexual reproduction by gametangial copulation. Sexual spores zygospores.
Higher Fungi	Ascomycotina (Ascomycetes)	Mycelium septate or single cells (yeasts) Asexual spores (conidia) borne exogenously. Sexual spores (ascospores) borne within sac or ascus; usually 8 in number. Asci may be borne singly or in groups within a fruiting body (ascocarp).
	Basidiomycotina (Basidiomycetes)	Mycelium septate or single cells (yeasts) Asexual spores, if formed, exogenous. Sexual spores (basidiospores) borne exogenously on a basidium — often within macroscopic fruiting body (basidiocarp).
	Deuteromycotina (Fungi Imperfecti)	Mycelium septate* or single cells (yeasts) Asexual spores borne exogenously, sometimes within pycnidium. Sexual reproduction not known.

* coenocytic mycelial fungi without a sexual phase are classified in Lower Fungi.

† Ainsworth G C 1973 In: Ainsworth G C, Sussman A S (eds) The fungi: an advanced treatise, vol 4a. Academic Press, London

Chapter Two FUNGAL PATHOGENS OF MAN AND ANIMALS

Only some 180 of the very large number of fungal species, estimates vary from 100 000 to 250 000, are capable of causing disease (mycosis) in man and animals by tissue invasion. However, the number of causal agents does not relate to the incidence or importance of these diseases which account for considerable morbidity and some mortality. Dermatophyte infections of the feet and yeast infections of the mouth and vagina occur almost as frequently as the common cold, and each year, in the southwest USA, some 12 000 infections that require medical attention and about 80 deaths are caused by a single fungus *Coccidioides immitis*.

The diseases caused by fungi can be divided into three broad groups; superficial mycoses, affecting the keratinous tissues of the skin, hair and nail and the mucous membranes; subcutaneous mycoses, which involve the skin, subcutaneous tissues and bone and show slow localized spread; systemic mycoses, usually initiated in the lung and sometimes becoming widely disseminated. There is considerable variation in the pathogenicity of the causal fungi. Some systemic fungal pathogens such as *C. immitis* and *Histoplasma capsulatum*, are highly pathogenic and capable of establishing an infection in all exposed individuals (true pathogens), others such as *Candida albicans* and *Aspergillus fumigatus* are opportunistic pathogens and in general they cause disease only in a host that has been predisposed physically or physiologically by an underlying disease or by treatment of that disease with, for example, cytotoxic or immunosuppressive drugs.

Although the species of causal fungus is important, in some mycoses the type and severity of an infection is largely dependent on the degree of exposure to the fungus, the site and method of entry into the body, as well as the immunological competence of the host.

Superficial infections of the keratinized tissues (ringworm) usually result from the transfer of fungus-infected keratin, directly or indirectly, from the infected to the uninfected; mucous membrane infections result from a localized change in the resistance of the host tissue, allowing infection by a commensal fungus. Subcutaneous infections result from the inoculation to the cutaneous and subcutaneous tissues of fungi growing as saprophytes in soil and decaying vegetation. Systemic infections are usually caused by soil fungi which produce large numbers of airborne spores, the size of which, if inhaled, allows them to penetrate deep into the respiratory system and initiate the primary pulmonary disease. Rarely, a systemic infection may be caused by a fungus which is a recognized subcutaneous pathogen, or subcutaneous disease may result from direct inoculation to these tissues of fungi usually associated with systemic or superficial infections.

In general, therefore, the mycoses are not contagious and are usually contracted from exogenous sources. The notable and important exception is ringworm for which the majority of causal fungi, although easily cultivated on artificial media, are hardly known to occur naturally except as agents of disease. Infections due to *Candida* species also differ in that they are usually endogenous in origin.

Some fungal pathogens have a strictly limited distribution, for example, *C. immitis* occurs only in the soil of southwest USA and parts of South America. Others have a much wider distribution although they may occur predominantly in certain regions; *H. capsulatum* is found mainly in the Mississippi and Ohio river valleys in the USA but occurs also in many other parts of the world. Local variations also occur, usually because of specific properties of soils such as enrichment by faecal material, exemplified by the close association of *Cryptococcus neoformans* with bird droppings and the prevalence of *H.*

capsulatum in caves inhabited by bats and in the soil of old chicken runs.

The incidence of all the mycoses, however, is directly related to those factors which affect the degree of exposure to the causal fungi such as living conditions and occupational and leisure activities. Systemic mycoses occur most frequently in workers in agriculture or the construction industries following disturbance of soils containing the causal fungi. Field workers in warm climates, particularly in regions where thorny vegetation is common, who wear little protective clothing frequently contract subcutaneous infections following minor injuries. Animal ringworm is an occupational hazard for farmers, veterinarians and others closely associated with animals. Ringworm of the feet (athlete's foot), with associated infections of nails and groin, commonly occurs in competitive swimmers, sportsmen and industrial workers because of their regular use of communal bathing facilities.

The mycoses are not notifiable diseases and their true incidence is unknown, but it is recognized that they are grossly under-reported and represent a much greater health problem than is generally realized. In Britain, during one year, foot ringworm was considered to be responsible for the loss of 110 000 working man-days in the mining industry alone and it has been estimated that approximately 250 000 new ringworm infections occur in this country each year. In the USA the annual expenditure on ringworm medications is reported to be in the region of 25 million dollars and around 9 million dollars is spent on treatment of the many thousands of new cases of coccidioidomycoses that occur each year and which are believed to account for nearly a million lost working days.

The incidence of opportunistic infections with, for example, *Aspergillus* and *Candida* has increased greatly following the wide-spread use of antibiotics and immunosuppressive drugs and the introduction of new surgical procedures. In transplant surgery these two fungi are among the most frequent causes of failure due to infection.

Like other microbial infections, diagnosis of the mycoses depends upon the recognition of the pathogen in tissue by direct microscopy, by isolation of the causal fungus in culture or by the detection of specific immunological changes in the host. The mycoses may mimic a number of other diseases and clinical signs, symptoms and radiological investigations are usually of very limited value for diagnosis.

In addition to causing infection, fungi may cause allergic disease in man, usually affecting the lungs and nasal passages following inhalation of fungal spores. Fungi may also cause serious, sometimes fatal, toxic effects, either following ingestion of poisonous mushrooms/toadstools (mycetismus) or the consumption of mouldy foodstuffs which contain toxic, fungal secondary metabolites (mycotoxicosis).

Chapter Three IMMUNITY TO FUNGAL INFECTIONS

Our knowledge of immunity to fungal infections is more restricted than for bacterial and virus infections. We do know, however, that infection (even subclinical) with certain pathogens confers lifelong immunity. It is also clear that immune deficiencies predispose to infection with both established and opportunistic fungal pathogens and that for a number of established pathogens genetic differences predispose the more severe disseminated forms of the disease.

MECHANISMS OF IMMUNITY

Immunity to infection involves both the non-specific (innate) and specific (acquired) immune responses. The two categories of response are to a considerable extent intertwined and interdependent; phagocytic cells (neutrophils, monocytes, macrophages) and T and B lymphocytes are believed to function together in protecting the host but the exact extent to which each is involved is not known and in any case this will differ with the individual and for different types of infection.

In fungal infections, non-specific factors have an important role in primary defence. Passive protection is provided by intact skin and mucosal surfaces which are generally considered to be resistant to infection. Fatty acids in sebum also provide protection because of their antifungal activity and serum has a similar inhibitory effect on a number of fungal pathogens. Within living tissues, however, it is the active, non-specific immune responses involving phagocytic cells which are of major importance and capable of effectively dealing with the intrusion of small numbers of fungal cells. Alveolar macrophages, for example, are important in engulfing cells in the lungs which are then removed by ciliary action and coughing. Similarly macrophages in the liver and spleen can remove fungi from the bloodstream. However, it is clear from a number of investigations that T lymphocytes in conjunction with monocytes play the most important role in protecting against fungal pathogens and it is known that a large proportion of individuals with serious fungal infections have functional T cell defects. The role of the B lymphocyte in protecting the host is less clear and for the mycoses the B cell is not thought to be as important as that of the T cell. Immunoglobulins of all classes are produced in infection, with the precise antibody response depending on the pathogen, host and type of infection. These antibody responses are extremely useful in the diagnosis of infections but evidence of the protective effect of antibody is fragmentary and in experimental work only partial protection has been observed by transfer of specific antibody. Specific antibody on the surface of fungal cells will assist in phagocytosis by facilitating attachment of neutrophils and macrophages, which have Fc receptor sites on their surface, but direct antibody-mediated killing of fungi has not been fully confirmed. However, it has been shown that antibody enables monocytes to kill *Cryptococcus neoformans* by a non-phagocytic mechanism. The precise extent to which complement is involved as an opsonin in phagocytic killing of fungi is also unclear. With *Candida* the C_3 component of complement activated by the alternative pathway has been directly implicated in phagocytic killing but it is not known if this commonly occurs with other fungal pathogens.

Microbial factors that facilitate infections by damaging of neutralizing host responses and which have been found in bacterial infections, have been little studied in fungal infections but it is thought that many fungal pathogens, particularly opportunistic pathogens such as *Candida* exploit deficiencies in the immune system rather than create susceptibility by regulating the immunological response. However, the importance of the various fungal antigens in the disease process has yet to be elucidated. It is possible that some antigens, perhaps depending on their mode of presentation may cause anergy.

DEFECTS IN THE IMMUNE RESPONSE

Opportunistic fungal pathogens exploit impaired defences in those in whom non-specific and specific mechanisms of resistance are diminished. True pathogens also cause infections more frequently in such individuals, who are also more likely to develop disseminated disease.

In some cases, the immune deficiencies that predispose to fungal infection are acquired congenitally and are associated with thymic defects, for example, in patients with chronic mucocutaneous candidosis. In most instances, however, fungal infections arise in patients with immune defects resulting from an underlying disease such as malignancy, from the treatment of that disease with cytotoxic or immunosuppressive drugs or from the use of these agents in transplantation surgery.

The principal defects that arise are a gross reduction in the number of neutrophils (neutropenia) and/or defects in neutrophil function. These occur mainly in those with haematological malignances, whether untreated or treated with cytotoxic agents or with irradiation prior to bone marrow transplantation. Defects in T and B cell function are also of prime importance and these may occur in certain types of haematological malignancy and in patients with particular forms of solid tumours. Again the treatment of these conditions has a profound effect on the lymphocytic response, particularly that of the T cell response which may be eliminated for long periods depending on the drugs used and the dosage and duration of therapy. Adrenocortical steroids, for example, reduce the numbers of circulating T and B cells and affect almost all of their functions.

There is considerable scope for further studies in the area of immunity to fungal infections and it is likely that a proper understanding of the mechanisms involved will await further work on the pathogenesis of fungal disease and further knowledge of immunology in general.

Chapter Four
DIAGNOSIS OF THE MYCOSES

As for other microbial infections the diagnosis of the mycoses depends upon a combination of clinical observation and laboratory investigation. Laboratory procedures include culture of the fungus, its recognition in the tissue by direct examination and the detection of specific humoral and/or cell mediated responses using a variety of serological methods, skin tests and in vitro tests of lymphocyte sensitization. The precise value of each of these components varies with the type of infection and the causal fungus.

The details of the media and procedures referred to in this chapter are given in the Appendix.

CLINICAL DIAGNOSIS

Clinical criteria give only a presumptive diagnosis of fungal infection. Superficial and subcutaneous mycoses often produce characteristic lesions which strongly suggest their fungal aetiology but they may also closely resemble other diseases. Moreover, it is not unusual to find that the appearance of lesions has been considerably modified and rendered atypical by previous therapy with, for example, topical steroids.

With the systemic mycoses there are no signs or symptoms which specifically indicate fungal disease and, since early diagnosis considerably increases the chances of successful treatment, it is important that the possibility of fungal involvement should be considered from the outset. Fortunately, within recent years, the importance of the mycoses has been better recognized and this, together with modern techniques for patient evaluation, has improved the accuracy and speed of diagnosis. For example, echocardiography has been used to demonstrate fungal vegetations on heart valves and the usefulness of examination of the eyes for endophthalmitis, a common complication of systemic candidosis, is now established.

LABORATORY DIAGNOSIS

Role of the laboratory

Laboratory procedures may confirm a clinical diagnosis, establish a fungal cause in a disease of unknown aetiology or exclude fungal involvement where there are several possible diagnoses. When a diagnosis of fungal infection has been established the laboratory may assist with the choice of therapeutic agents, monitoring the course of the disease and confirming mycological cure. In some instances, for example with the opportunistic mycoses, the laboratory may be able to provide only subjective evidence to be considered along with the clinical findings and in such cases close liaison between the clinician and the laboratory worker is particularly necessary.

It is important that the laboratory receives the correct type of specimen together with adequate clinical data so that the appropriate investigations can be carried out. Information on factors such as travel or residence abroad, animal contacts and the occupation of the patient will enable the laboratory to direct or modify their procedures towards a particular fungus or group of fungi when appropriate.

Types of specimen

Superficial mycoses

In skin infections a fungal lesion usually spreads outwards in a concentric fashion with healing in the central region. Material should therefore be collected by scraping outwards from the edges of the lesions with a scalpel blade; when there is minimal scaling as, for example, with lesions of the glabrous skin, it is preferable and sometimes necessary to use Sellotape to remove adequate material for examination.

Specimens from the scalp are best obtained by scraping with a blunt scalpel so that the sample includes hair stubs, contents of plugged follicles and scales. Hairs which have been cut rather than plucked are seldom satisfactory. Wood's light (p. 60) may be used to detect scalp ringworm or to select material for culture when the infection is caused by species which produce fluorescence of infected hair.

Ringworm of the scalp, especially if caused by anthropophilic species may cause minimal lesions which are difficult to detect clinically. Infections of this type when caused by dermatophyte species which produce fluorescence of infected hair can usually be detected by Wood's light. Otherwise the use of the hairbrush sampling technique to obtain cultures is recommended. This involves thoroughly brushing the scalp and using the hairbrush (or scalp massage pad) to inoculate petri-dishes of isolation media. Nail specimens should be clipped from the free edge, taken as far back in the nail as possible and should include its full thickness. Fungus in the distal portion of the nail is often non-viable and if culture does fail for this reason success can sometimes be obtained by culturing 'borings' taken from nearer the base of the nail.

In all cases, cleaning the site with surgical spirit before taking the specimen may be helpful and should always be done if greasy ointments or if powders have been used for treatment. Material is best collected into folded squares of paper which, by permitting drying of the specimen, reduces bacterial contamination and also provides conditions under which specimens may be stored for long periods without appreciable loss in viability of ringworm fungi.

For mucous membrane infections also, scrapings are preferable to swabs. If swabs are used for sampling they are best sent to the laboratory in transport medium since yeasts rapidly lose viability in dry swabs.

Subcutaneous mycoses

Scrapings or crusts from the superficial parts of

subcutaneous lesions may be satisfactory for microscopy and culture but contamination with bacteria and saprophytic fungi is common and aspirated samples of pus and/or biopsy specimens are much more valuable. Biopsy should, however, be avoided in suspected sporotrichosis since this may spread infection and hinder healing.

Systemic mycoses

Patients with suspected systemic mycoses should have specimens taken from as many sites as possible and it is important to ensure that specimens such as sputum and urine are freshly collected. Twenty-four-hour sputum samples, or urine samples from catheter bags, are unsatisfactory since yeasts multiply quite rapidly in such material. A catheter specimen of urine is best but failing this a midstream urine sample is usually satisfactory. Care should be taken not to overinterpret the high counts of yeasts often encountered in patients with an indwelling urinary catheter.

In patients with suspected pulmonary mycoses, sputum samples are useful, particularly in the case of infection with established fungal pathogens. However, interpretation of the results with opportunistic pathogens such as *Candida*, which may be present in sputum specimens simply as a result of oropharyngeal contamination, is much more difficult and here samples of bronchial secretions more accurately reflect the flora of the lung. It is often unclear whether the recovery of opportunistic fungi from sputum or bronchial secretions indicates tissue invasion or lung colonization and it may be necessary to use techniques such as bronchial brushing or lung biopsy to obtain material suitable for diagnosis.

Processing of specimens

Pretreatment of specimens is sometimes necessary or advisable before examination by microscopy and culture. Samples of cerebrospinal fluid (c.s.f.) and urine are best centrifuged and the deposit resuspended in a minimal volume of saline in order to detect the low numbers of fungi sometimes present. Sputum samples may also be centrifuged if they are first liquified by digestion in pancreatin.

It is often helpful and sometimes necessary to culture measured volumes of specimens. By estimating the number of viable fungal elements, expressed as the number of colony forming units (c.f.u.) per ml, the severity of an infection can be assessed and the result of therapy can be monitored from a series of specimens.

Direct examination

Potassium hydroxide mounts

The majority of specimens can be satisfactorily examined in wet mounts after partial digestion with 10–20% KOH. Representative portions of skin, hair and nail should be mounted under a coverslip in KOH on a microscope slide; this will clear the material within 5–20 minutes, depending on its thickness, and allow recognition of fungal structures. Warming over a low flame, for example the pilot light of a bunsen-burner, hastens the digestion of the keratin but care must be taken to avoid crystallization of the KOH. Specimens of sputum, centrifuged c.s.f. or urine deposits may be examined without prior preparation but it is nevertheless better to mix samples with equal volumes of KOH to clear the host cellular debris.

The ability to differentiate between fungal structures and naturally occurring artefacts develops with experience. The fungi can be stained, for example, by adding Parker Quink ink (50% v/v) to 20% KOH but the advantages of this are minimal as artefacts also take up the stain.

The small size of *Histoplasma* yeast cells makes them difficult to detect and KOH mounts are unsatisfactory. For suspected histoplasmosis, Giemsa stained smears of sputum, pus, biopsies, etc. are advised.

Histopathology

There is no tissue reaction which is typical of a fungal infection. In superficial infection the histopathological picture presented is that of an acute, subacute or chronic dermatitis with folliculitis in inflammatory lesions of hairy skin. In subcutaneous and systemic infections a granulomatous reaction, often with fibrosis or pyogenic inflammation is usual, the reaction varying according to the site and evolution of the condition. With *Cryptococcus neoformans* there is characteristically little tissue response. Diagnosis therefore depends on the demonstration of fungi within the tissues. Haematoxylin and eosin (HE) staining is seldom of value for the detection of fungal elements in tissue sections and therefore specific fungal stains, such as periodic acid-Schiff (PAS), Grocott-Gomori methenamine-silver and Gridley are widely used for this purpose. In addition Mayer's mucicarmine is used specifically to demonstrate the capsular material of *Cr. neoformans*. The causal agents of phycomycosis are unusual among pathogenic fungi in that they do not stain with PAS and are usually visible in HE stained material.

In the case of infections with dematiaceous fungi the dark brown colour of the hyphae renders them relatively easy to see and although special stains are not strictly required, PAS staining of some of the sections is usually helpful.

Fluorescent-antibody staining

Fluorescent-antibody staining may be used to demonstrate fungi in material such as pus, blood, c.s.f., tissue-impression smears and in paraffin sections of formalin-fixed tissue; it is less satisfactory for sputum samples. The main advantage of this technique lies in its ability to detect fungus when there are only a few elements present, as for example in pus from *Sporothrix schenckii* infections. Its use, however, is limited by the restricted availability of the specific antisera required.

Culture

With very few exceptions the isolation of pathogenic fungi is not difficult, the essential requirement being an organic source of nitrogen in the isolation medium. Broth media are not recommended and the agar media commonly used are Sabouraud's dextrose and 4% malt extract. These media may be supplemented with antibiotics, such as chloramphenicol (0.05 g/l), to minimize bacterial contamination and cycloheximide (Actidione; 0.5 g/l) to reduce contamination with saprophytic fungi. Cycloheximide should not be used in attempts to isolate *Cryptococcus, Histoplasma, Aspergillus* or *Hendersonula* as these fungi are sensitive to this antibiotic. Special media may be used for isolation and to assist with rapid identification when the identity of a particular pathogen is strongly suspected or known. For example, *Cr. neoformans* develops as brown colonies on Niger seed or caffeic acid/ferric citrate agar.

Many fungal pathogens have an optimum growth temperature below 37 °C. Isolation from suspected superficial mycoses is usually attempted by incubating cultures at 25–30 °C. For subcutaneous and systemic mycoses cultures are usually incubated at this lower temperature and also at 37 °C. With certain dimorphic pathogens such as *Histoplasma capsulatum* and *Blastomyces dermatitidis* the mycelial phase develops on the commonly used isolation media at 25–30 °C and the yeast phase of the organism develops at 37 °C on rich media, such as brain-heart infusion or blood-agar. Fungi develop relatively slowly and cultures should be retained for at least 3 weeks and in some cases up to 6 weeks before being discarded. In many instances, however, positive results are obtained within 7–10 days and *Aspergillus* and *Candida* species, for example, usually develop within 24–72 hours. Cultures should therefore be examined for growth at regular intervals and subcultures made from developing colonies of suspected pathogens if these are threatened by overgrowth of saprophytic contaminants.

Specimens may be cultured on agar media in petri-dishes or test-tube slants but petri-dish cultures should *not* be used for the isolation of systemic pathogens such as *H. capsulatum* or *Coccidioides immitis* because of the serious risk of infection; these fungi should always be handled in a safety cabinet. If screw-cap containers are used then caps should not be fully tightened since lack of oxygen will inhibit fungal development. Blood cultures should be taken into vented, biphasic (broth/agar slant) blood culture bottles; special media are not required and blood culture systems used for the isolation of aerobic bacteria are satisfactory for growth of pathogenic fungi.

Interpretation of culture results

The significance of a fungal isolate depends on its source and identity. The isolation of established pathogens such as *H. capsulatum* or *C. immitis* from any specimen is generally regarded as evidence of infection with these fungi. However, with opportunistic pathogens such as *Candida* or *Aspergillus* the situation is not as clear cut. Isolation of these fungi from normally sterile sites, from blood cultures, c.s.f. or pleural fluid usually provides reliable evidence of infection but when they are recovered from material such as pus, sputum or urine the results must be interpreted with care. Attention should be given, for example, to the quantity of fungus isolated and further investigations undertaken.

It should be remembered that many species of fungi may cause disease in severely immunocompromised individuals and no isolate from this type of patient should be lightly discarded as a contaminant.

Identification of fungal isolates

The identification of a mycelial fungus involves a detailed study of its macroscopic and microscopic morphology and since its morphology can vary with the medium and growth temperature, it may be necessary to study isolates on a range of media at several temperatures.

After noting the macroscopic features of the colony, such as the colour and texture of growth, slide mounts should be made in lactophenol-cotton blue for microscopical examination; it may be necessary to make several preparations, perhaps over a period of time, in order to see characteristic structures on which an identification can be based. If delicate sporing structures are disrupted when mounts are made, special techniques such as slide culture, which allow fungal growth to be examined undisturbed should be used.

Biochemical rather than morphological criteria are used for the identification of yeasts but certain morphological features remain important and these include cell shape, size, presence or absence of capsules, ability to produce mycelium or pseudomycelium, mode of asexual reproduction (budding, fission) and the method of sexual reproduction. The important biochemical criteria are the ability to assimilate certain carbon (mainly sugars) and nitrogen compounds and to ferment sugars.

Identification of yeasts can involve the use of a wide range of carbon compounds and certain other quite involved investigational procedures. However, the identification of medically important yeasts can usually be satisfactorily achieved with a more limited range of tests and furthermore for the most frequently encountered yeast pathogens a number of special tests have been evolved. For example, two tests are available for the rapid identification of *C. albicans*, namely, the production of germ tubes in serum after 1–2 hours incubation of 37 °C, and the production of chlamydospores under microaerophilic conditions on special media such as Czapek-Dox+Tween 80 agar. Special media containing niger seed (*Guizotia abyssinica*) extract or caffeic acid/ferric citrate are also now widely used for the rapid identification of *Cr. neoformans* which develops as brown/black colonies on these substrates.

Commercial kits for the identification of medically important yeasts by their assimilation patterns are now widely available. They are convenient to use and give results which are comparable in accuracy to those obtained by the above procedures.

Immunology and serology

The specific immune response that results from exposure to cell wall, cytoplasmic or extracellular fungal antigens during fungal infection can be used for diagnosis and also by monitoring this response the prognosis and the result of therapy can be assessed. Skin tests and in vitro lymphocyte stimulation tests are used to detect cell mediated changes and serological tests to detect humoral antibody production and/or the presence of fungal antigens in body fluids.

The type of immune response depends on the fungus involved, the form of the disease and the immunological competence of the host.

Cell mediated tests

Skin tests. Individuals who become infected with, for

example, *Histoplasma* or *Coccidioides* develop a delayed type IV hypersensitivity reaction within 1–14 days and this persists for many years. This sensitization can be demonstrated by skin tests in which a reaction (induration/erythema) occurs 24–72 hours following intradermal inoculation of the appropriate fungal extract or culture filtrate. In endemic areas a large proportion of the population may be skin test positive and as a consequence skin testing is more useful for epidemiological work than for diagnosis since a positive reaction is more likely to indicate previous rather than current disease. Their diagnostic usefulness is also limited by the cross-reactivity which can occur because of common antigens shared by the major fungal pathogens. For this reason it is preferable to test simultaneously with antigens from several fungi so that the relative strength of reaction to each can be compared.

Positive skin tests usually revert to negative in those with severe or disseminated disease and so may be used as prognostic indicators. Negative skin test results may also be obtained when there is no infection, infection is at an early stage and in those with defective cellular immunity. In lung hypersensitivity diseases skin tests are very useful for diagnosis. In this case, type I (immediate) and/or type III (arthus) reactions, associated with reaginic IgE antibodies occur.

Table 4.2 shows the mycoses for which skin tests are useful for diagnosis.

In vitro tests. In vitro tests to demonstrate acquired hypersensitivity, such as those for macrophage migration-inhibition and blast formation of sensitized lymphocytes in the presence of specific fungal antigens, are being used increasingly for the diagnosis of fungal disease.

Serological tests

Antibody detection. Serological tests for antibody detection are of value only for the diagnosis of systemic and subcutaneous mycoses. They may also be used to assess prognosis and response to therapy. For some diseases the tests are reliable but for others they provide only presumptive evidence of infection and results must be considered along with other clinical and laboratory findings. In certain cases there is a need to improve specificity and some patients may have antibodies in the absence of infection because they have been previously exposed to the fungus either as a saprophyte or as a commensal. Tests may also lack sensitivity; some infected patients may have little or no detectable antibody response because their infection is at an early stage or because of underlying disease or chemotherapy.

For some diseases, cross-reactions which occur because of the complex and crude nature of certain fungal antigenic extracts also cause problems with the interpretation of results. Unfortunately the most unsatisfactory tests are those for the opportunistic systemic mycoses which are among the most difficult to diagnose by other means. For these infections, a series of tests is more helpful than a single investigation since in general, a high or rapidly rising antibody titre is indicative of infection.

The techniques used for the detection of antibodies and in some cases antigen, are essentially those used elsewhere in medical microbiology (Table 4.1) to detect agglutinating, precipitating and complement-fixing antibodies belonging to the IgA, IgG and IgM subclasses of immunoglobulins. The predominant class of antibody produced depends on the host, the fungus and the type of infection, whereas the technique determines the class of immunoglobulin and the type of antibody detected.

Table 4.1 Serological tests used in mycology

Agglutination	— whole cell (WCA), inert particle: usually latex (LPA) or passive haemagglutination (PHA)
Immunodiffusion (ID)	
Counter-immunoelectrophoresis (CIE)	
Complement fixation (CF)	
Indirect fluorescent antibody (IFA)	
Enzyme-linked immunosorbent assay (ELISA)	
Radioimmunoassay (RIA) — solid phase, competitive	

Until recently the most widely used test was ID in agar or agarose for the detection of fungal precipitins and it was used as a primary screening test even when more sensitive tests were available. However, CIE has now gained almost universal acceptance as a more rapid and sensitive method of demonstrating precipitins to fungi and it also offers a more convenient way of determining precipitin titres. More sensitive tests such as ELISA and RIA are now being introduced for antibody detection but in some cases, for example in candidosis, increased sensitivity is not necessarily an advantage.

Table 4.2 shows the most widely used serological tests for diagnosis of the various mycoses. Many of these are commercially available as serodiagnostic kits.

Table 4.2 Immunological and serological tests commonly used for diagnosis of fungal infections

Disease	Test	Comments
Aspergillosis	Skin	Useful in allergic disease only
	ID, CIE	Detection of precipitins useful in all forms of disease. Used also for antigen detection — low sensitivity
	ELISA, RIA	Useful for antibody and antigen detection — offer improved sensitivity
Blastomycosis	Skin	Limited value, negative in *ca.* 50% active cases
	ID, CIE	Precipitins detectable in <80% cases. Negative result does not preclude infection
	CF	Negative result of no value. Titre ⩾ 1:8 taken as positive. High or rapidly rising titre more significant. Value limited by cross-reactions with other mycoses
Systemic candidosis	Skin	Of no diagnostic value, positive in immunologically competent individuals. Used to detect anergy
	ID, CIE	Precipitins may indicate disease or colonization but in infection tendency for higher or rising titres. Negative results in anergic patients. Cytoplasmic antigens give best specificity
	WCA	Agglutinins — as for precipitins. Same drawbacks, also less specific
	LPA, IFA, PHA	Less widely used, lack specificity. LPA also used for antigen detection
	ELISA, RIA	Used for both antigen and antibody detection
Coccidioidomycosis	Skin	Indicates past or recent infection. Epidemiological tool, little diagnostic value — negative in disseminated disease
	ID, CIE	Useful for indicating early infection. Precipitins short-lived. Negative reaction does not preclude infection. Tube precipitation test method also used
	LPA	Similar results to precipitin tests — less specific

Table 4.2 Cont'd

Disease	Test	Comments
	CF	Most useful for diagnosis of disseminated disease. Negative does not preclude infection. Rising/falling titres of prognostic value. Tests on c.s.f. helpful for diagnosis of meningeal infection
		Use of precipitin and CF tests in combination gives positive results in < 90% cases. Some cross-reactions with histoplasmosis and blastomycosis
Cryptococcosis	WCA	Used to detect antibody titre. False positives occur, *approx.* 95% specific. Negative does not preclude infection.
	IFA	For antibody detection. Less specific (approx. 80%) than WCA. Negative result does not preclude infection.
	LPA	Most useful. Detects capsular antigen, usually in serum, c.s.f. Good specificity and approx. 90% sensitivity. Rising/falling titres of prognostic value
	CIE	May also be used to detect antigen
Histoplasmosis	Skin	Indicates past or recent infection — epidemiological tool. Not recommended for diagnosis — induces humoral antibody response which confuses interpretation of serology results
	CF	Uses histoplasmin (mycelial phase culture filtrate) or killed whole yeast cells (YP). Positive results in < 96% cases. YP antibodies appear first and best for screening active cases. Histoplasmin antibodies occur later, more elevated in chronic forms. Negative results do not preclude infection. Titre changes of prognostic value. Some cross-reactions
	ID, CIE	Useful screening test. Positive in < 85% cases. Fewer cross-reactions than CF. Positive results should be confirmed by CF test
	LPA	Useful for diagnosis of acute disease. Negative results possible in chronic histoplasmosis. Less useful than ID and CF
Mycetoma	ID, CIE	Not usually necessary for diagnosis but useful for distinguishing between eumycetoma and actinomycetoma when cultures are negative
Paracoccidiodomycosis	Skin	Unreliable. Negative in many with advanced disease and cross-reactions common
	ID, CIE	Precipitins of diagnostic and prognostic value. Positive in < 95% cases. Good specificity
	CF	Useful for diagnosis. Positive in < 80% cases. Highest titres in pulmonary and disseminated disease. Some cross-reaction with histoplasmosis
Sporotrichosis	Skin	Not fully developed. Problems with specificity
	LPA	Useful, specific and sensitive (< 90% cases)
	WCA	Comparable sensitivity to LPA, some false positives in patients with leishmaniasis

Antigen detection. Tests for the detection of antibodies are of limited value in the early stages of infection and in patients with impaired immunity. In such cases serological tests for the detection of fungal antigens are of particular value. The diagnosis of cryptococcosis using an LPA test for the detection of capsular antigen in c.s.f. and other body fluids is well established.

Tests are now being introduced for the detection of *Aspergillus* and *Candida* antigens, mainly for the diagnosis of serious systemic infections in severely immunocompromised patients such as those undergoing bone marrow transplants. Because of the low levels of circulating antigen present in infected individuals, the tests need to be extremely sensitive and although ID and CIE have been used for antigen detection, the most promising results have been obtained with more sensitive techniques such as ELISA and RIA. The antigen detection tests available for diagnosis are included in Table 4.2.

New approaches to the detection of fungi

Gas liquid chromatography (GLC)

Various forms of this technique, now widely used for the diagnosis of anaerobic infections, are being examined for possible use in the diagnosis of systemic fungal infections. GLC has shown that patients with systemic candidosis have raised arabinitol and mannose levels and abnormal GLC peak patterns have also been detected in the sera of patients with *Candida* septicaemia. Electron-capture GLC of c.s.f. samples from patients with cryptococcal meningitis also show characteristic profiles. These features may eventually prove of value for diagnosis.

Chapter Five
TREATMENT OF THE MYCOSES

The development of drugs for the treatment of the mycoses has lagged considerably behind that for bacterial infections. This is largely because fungi, like man and animals, are eukaryotic and substances which will kill or inhibit growth of a fungal pathogen will usually also have a toxic effect on host tissues. Those antifungals that can be used therapeutically usually exploit the minor differences in the sterol composition of the cell membranes which in animals is cholesterol and in fungi is mainly ergosterol. Strangely, it has not yet been possible to find an antifungal which selectively affects the fungal cell wall, the most obvious structural difference between animal and fungal cells.

GENERAL ASPECTS OF THERAPY

Most clinically useful antifungal drugs are primarily fungistatic and any fungicidal activity which they possess occurs only at high concentrations or after prolonged exposure. Fungi are also able to adapt physiologically and morphologically to combat adverse environmental conditions and for these reasons the concentration of drug that can be achieved in tissue and the period of time during which this can be maintained is of considerably more importance than is the case for antibacterial drugs.

There is no direct relationship between the in vitro activity of an antifungal drug and its clinical efficacy.

Eradication of a fungal pathogen may result from the effect of diverse factors such as adverse growth conditions in tissues and/or host defence mechanisms, combining with the antifungal drug at a concentration considerably less than the in vitro minimum inhibitory concentration (m.i.c.) for the fungus concerned. Conversely, the ability of a fungus to adapt to a resistant growth form means that prolonged exposure may be necessary or the tissue concentration of a drug may need to be higher than the in vitro m.i.c. of the vegetative phase if a cure is to be obtained. The mode of action of the various drugs on a susceptible fungus is also important and this may vary considerably. Some drugs, such as polyene antibiotics, have little effect at low concentrations but cause growth to cease sharply at the m.i.c. Others, such as griseofulvin and the imidazole drugs are active at very low concentrations and gradually reduce the rate of growth as the concentration rises until it ceases entirely at the m.i.c.

There is considerable variation in the spectrum of activity of antifungal drugs, from extremely narrow for griseofulvin, with activity only against dermatophytes, to the broad spectrum of amphotericin B with activity against almost all fungal pathogens. Although some isolates of a particular species may vary slightly in sensitivity to a drug, gross variation in sensitivity is unusual and neither naturally occurring resistance nor development of resistance is the major problem it is with bacterial pathogens. This means that once the spectrum of activity of an antifungal has been established it can be selected for use in treatment according to the identity of the infecting fungus without the need to ascertain the sensitivity of a particular isolate. A notable exception in this respect is flucytosine to which primary and developed (secondary) resistance occurs relatively frequently and sensitivity testing of isolates prior to and during treatment is always necessary. For other drugs, although measurement of sensitivity is advisable when there is a failure to obtain the expected therapeutic response, experience has shown that drug resistance is extremely unlikely and that such failures usually result from factors such as malabsorption or antagonism by other concomitantly administered drugs.

Although the treatment of a number of mycotic infections is still far from satisfactory and presents a significant challenge in management, there is now a sufficient number of drugs and overlap between their spectrum of activity to allow some degree of selection for the treatment of most of the mycoses, subject of course to such limitations as may be posed by a particular patient or site of infection.

TOPICAL THERAPY

Local application of ointments, creams and lotions is used extensively in the treatment of superficial mycoses and is often the treatment of choice. Toxicity is not a problem since there is seldom penetration of significant amounts of drug into deeper tissue. However, contact dermatitis is an easily induced reaction and, despite their potent antifungal activity, the use of certain substances such as phenolic or mercuric compounds must be avoided.

A major defect of topical preparations is their inability to penetrate the keratin barrier and, although there may be quite significant differences in the in vitro activity of the antifungal agents they contain, the differences in their therapeutic efficacy are marginal. Keratolytic agents were included in many of the early topical preparations but this approach did not solve the problem. Such progress as has been made in the development of topical antifungals has been mainly in the production of preparations which are cosmetically more acceptable.

Topical therapy is most valuable for mucosal infections, for sites with a thin keratin layer such as the glabrous body skin and for diseases such as pityriasis versicolor and tinea nigra in which the causal fungi are concentrated in the upper portion of the horny layer. It is of little value for infections of nails, scalp or sites with a thick horny layer when, as for ringworm, growth and development takes place at the base of the keratin.

SYSTEMIC THERAPY

Systemic administration of antifungal drugs is essential for the treatment of deepseated mycoses and, because it circumvents the keratin barrier, it is also the ideal method of therapy for superficial infections. Administration by the oral route is simplest and most satisfactory but, because of poor absorption or degradation in the gastrointestinal tract, some drugs must be given parenterally, usually intravenously (i.v.), to achieve the necessary level of activity in body tissues. Some differential distribution also occurs within the body and the efficacy of a drug may depend on the site of infection, perhaps being enhanced by selectively concentrating in one organ and requiring supplementation by local infusion at other sites.

Toxicity is a major problem and few systemically administered drugs are completely free from adverse side effects. However, these are usually reversible and in most instances there is a wide margin between the therapeutic dose and the occurrence of serious toxicity. When this is not so, careful monitoring together with adjustments to the dose and the period of administration can sometimes be made to suit the requirements of the individual patient.

COMBINATION THERAPY

The use of a combination of drugs may be advantageous if their activity is not impaired by antagonism. In some cases the level of activity achieved is greater than the additive effect of the components (synergism), usually because the action of one drug enables the other to exert an enhanced inhibitory effect, for example, by being able to enter the cell more easily because the plasma-membrane has been damaged by its partner. Even if the combined effect is merely additive, the use of a combination of drugs is helpful since it allows a toxic drug to be used at a lower dose level and, in addition, development of resistance is less likely to occur.

Of the various antifungal drug combinations investigated so far, only one has proved to be advantageous. The combination of flucytosine and amphotericin B has an additive or possibly synergistic effect on susceptible fungi and also has the advantage of allowing a reduction in the dose of amphotericin B and of counteracting the development of resistance to flucytosine. So far, combinations of imidazole drugs and amphotericin B have been found to be antagonistic.

PROPHYLAXIS

Prophylactic measures to reduce the risk of fungal infection are not widely practised except perhaps for opportunistic *Candida* infections in patients undergoing transplant or cardiac surgery or those receiving prolonged steroid or antibiotic therapy. In such groups the prevention of a build-up of *Candida* in the mouth and gastrointestinal tract by oral administration of nystatin, amphotericin B or ketoconazole has been shown to be highly beneficial in preventing serious *Candida* sepsis. For superficial mycoses it has been shown that the regular use of an antifungal foot powder will minimize the spread of foot ringworm in those who regularly use communal bathing facilities and that oral griseofulvin reduces the incidence of ringworm infection in soldiers at high risk during field warfare in the tropics.

A vaccine which protects against *Coccidioides immitis* infection has been developed and is currently being evaluated for use in certain groups such as servicemen transferred into the endemic region of coccidioidomycosis.

ANTIFUNGAL DRUGS

Polyene antibiotics

Amphotericin B, nystatin and natamycin are derived from *Streptomyces* spp. They act by selectively binding to fungal cell membranes, causing an increase in membrane permeability, leakage of cell constituents and ultimately cell death. They have a broad spectrum of activity against mycelial fungi and yeasts.

Nystatin/natamycin

These are suitable only for topical use. Nystatin is non-toxic and is also used orally for its local effect in the gastrointestinal tract.

Amphotericin B

This is probably the most useful of the antifungal drugs and it may be used topically in superficial infections as well as parenterally to treat a wide variety of systemic mycoses. It is usually given i.v. for systemic infections. Around 95% of the drug binds to plasma proteins and rapidly leaves the circulation. Because of poor penetration into body fluids such as cerebrospinal fluid (c.s.f.), concomitant intrathecal administration is required in central nervous system infections.

The major limitation of amphotericin B is its serious adverse effects, particularly its nephrotoxicity. These toxic effects may be minimized by slowly increasing the dose to therapeutic levels but this is not advised in life-threatening infections which should always be treated aggressively. Many of amphotericin B's unpleasant side effects can be alleviated by other drugs and increasingly it is being used in combination with flucytosine which allows smaller doses of amphotericin to be given and further reduces the problems of toxicity.

Parenteral amphotericin B therapy need not wait for sensitivity tests as resistance to polyenes is very rare. Routine estimations of serum levels are of no practical benefit but renal function and blood biochemistry should be monitored regularly.

Amphotericin B, despite its toxicity, has revolutionized the treatment and improved the prognosis for systemic fungal infections and it remains the treatment of choice in life-threatening infections.

Griseofulvin

This antibiotic, derived from various *Penicillium* species, has a narrow spectrum of activity and is primarily active against dermatophytes. Its mode of action is not precisely known but it is the only antifungal to cause gross distortion of fungal hyphae. It has also been reported to affect microtubule assembly and to inhibit nucleic acid synthesis.

Griseofulvin is a safe drug, with few and only minor side effects at the therapeutic dose and it is suitable for long term treatment. It becomes selectively concentrated in keratinized tissues where it inhibits fungal growth sufficiently to prevent the invasion of the newly formed keratin. The duration of treatment required depends therefore on the time taken for outgrowth of infected keratin; infections of skin and hair require considerably shorter periods of therapy (4–6 weeks) than may be required for nail infections (4–12 months).

Griseofulvin remains the treatment of choice for most ringworm infections particularly those of scalp and nail which do not respond to topical therapy.

Flucytosine (5-fluorocytosine)

Flucytosine is a synthetic antifungal, a fluorinated pyrimidine, which is primarily active against yeasts. It acts by interfering with nucleic acid synthesis. It is well absorbed after oral administration and blood levels of up to 100 mg/l are easily achieved without toxic effects; if necessary it may also be given i.v. Only a small proportion of the drug is protein bound and it is largely excreted unchanged in the urine. It penetrates well into body fluids such as c.s.f.

A major drawback is that primary resistance to flucytosine occurs in 20% of clinical isolates. Secondary resistance also frequently develops during treatment, particularly in isolates that were only weakly sensitive initially. Sensitivity testing with flucytosine before and at regular intervals during therapy is therefore essential. Furthermore, blood levels of flucytosime should be monitored in patients with impaired renal function as they may accumulate toxic levels of the drug.

The problem of resistance has reduced the clinical value of flucytosine and it should not be used alone to treat life-threatening infections. It is now most often used in combination with amphotericin B.

Imidazoles

The synthetic imidazole derivatives are recent additions to the range of antifungals and many have still to be fully evaluated. The clinical usefulness of clotrimazole, miconazole, econazole, isoconazole, bifonazole and ketoconazole is, however, already established.

All the imidazoles have a broad spectrum of

activity with only minor variations between them; some are also active against gram positive bacteria.

Their mode of action is complex. They are believed to block ergosterol synthesis (affecting membrane permeability) and interfere with oxidative enzymes causing a lethal accumulation of hydrogen peroxide in the cells.

Imidazoles are widely used in the treatment of superficial mycoses. All are available for topical use but ketoconazole may also be orally administered. Parenteral miconazole and oral ketoconazole have also been used, with varying success, to treat a number of subcutaneous and systemic fungal infections; although it has yet to be fully evaluated, ketoconazole looks the more promising. Instances of liver damage have, however, been reported following oral therapy with ketoconazole and this risk has to be weighed against the potential benefits of treatment. Patients receiving oral ketoconazole should be carefully monitored both clinically and biochemically.

Other drugs

Rifampicin

Used in the treatment of tuberculosis, rifampicin also shows some antifungal activity. It is orally administered and has been used on a limited scale, usually in combination with amphotericin B, to treat systemic yeast infections.

Potassium iodide

Given orally, potassium iodide is at present the drug of choice for the treatment of the chronic lymphocutaneous form of sporotrichosis and also for infections due to the zygomycete *Basidiobolus*. Its mode of action is unknown as it has no demonstrable inhibitory effect on the causal fungi in vitro.

Hydroxystilbamidine

Although largely replaced by amphotericin B, oral hydroxystilbamidine may be used to treat blastomycosis, particularly the chronic pulmonary form of the disease. It is useful in patients who cannot tolerate amphotericin B.

SUPERFICIAL MYCOSES

Chapter Six RINGWORM

(Synonyms: tinea; dermatophytosis)

Ringworm, a complex of diseases affecting the keratinous tissues of hair, nail and the horny layer of the skin, is caused by a group of closely related fungi commonly referred to as dermatophytes. In its various forms, ringworm occurs in all parts of the world and the prevalent type in any region is governed mainly by the habits and living conditions of the population. Although often considered to be a trivial disease, the psychological effects of ringworm infection may be considerable and because of its high morbidity it is a costly disease in terms of treatment and loss of working time.

CLINICAL FORMS

The symptoms and the appearance of the lesions vary considerably according to the site of infection and the species of infecting fungus. Typically the lesions are spreading with a well demarcated, raised, erythematous border and there is usually some degree of scaling and inflammation. The characteristic circular lesions, from which the name of the disease is derived, are usually seen only on glabrous skin (Figs 6.1–6.3) and on the scalp and beard. Lesions in body folds, such as the groin, tend to spread outwards from the flexures. In foot ringworm, infection is frequently restricted to the toe-clefts and is commonly associated with peeling and maceration.

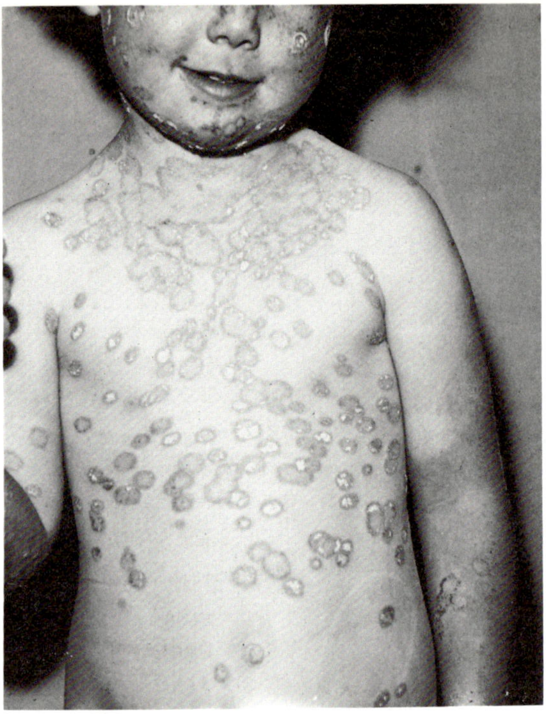

Fig. 6.1 Ringworm (Tinea corporis) in a child caused by *Microsporum canis* showing typical annular lesions with raised, scaling border and central healing

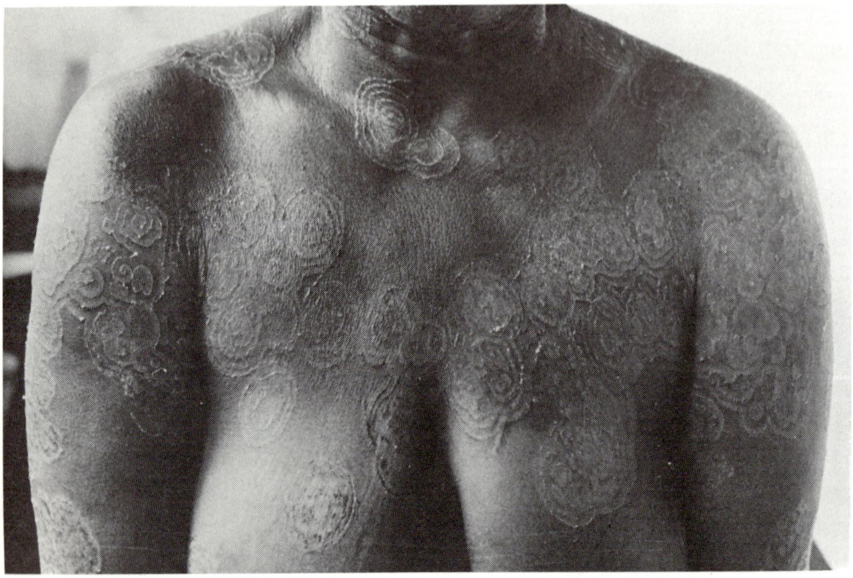

Fig. 6.2 Tinea imbricata (Tokelau) showing bizarre concentric pattern of raised scaly lesions. Native of Fiji

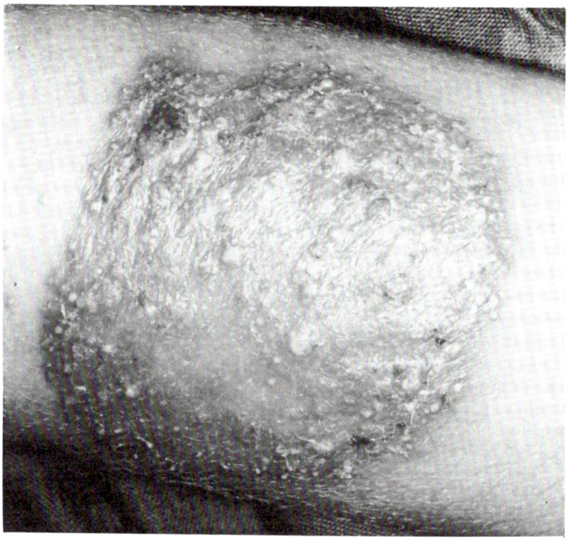

Fig. 6.3 Inflammatory ringworm lesion of the arm caused by *Trichophyton verrucosum*

Ringworm of the hand is often confined to the palm which may show only diffuse scaling. Nail infections are usually secondary to infections of the feet or hands; the nail becomes discoloured, thickened, raised and eventually friable (Fig. 6.4).

The host response is also very variable and ranges from slight skin scaling to a highly inflammatory,

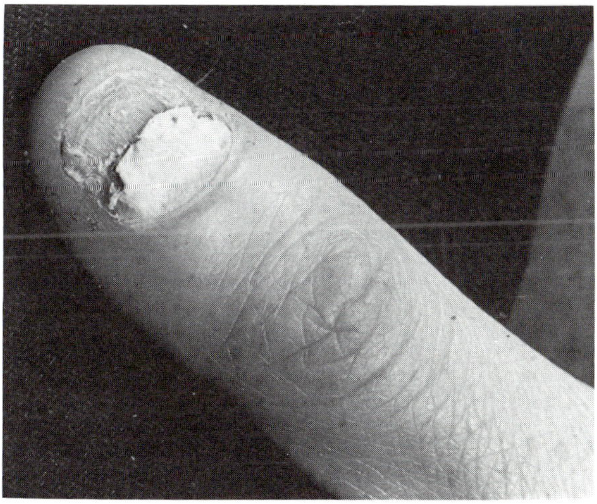

Fig. 6.4 Ringworm of nail (Tinea unguium) caused by *Trichophyton rubrum*

raised suppurating lesion called a kerion. In general, the inflammatory response is greatest when the scalp is involved and/or the causal dermatophyte is primarily a pathogen of animals. Scalp infections caused by anthropophilic dermatophytes are characteristically chronic and non-inflammatory. Three distinct clinical forms of scalp ringworm can be recognized depending upon the method by which the causal species invades the hair (Fig. 6.5). In one group of species, exemplified by *T. tonsurans* and *T. violaceum*, fungal growth and arthrospore production occurs entirely within the hair shaft (endothrix) and the hair is so weakened that it breaks off at, or below the mouth of the follicle which then becomes plugged with dirt and sebum to give what is described clinically as 'black dot' ringworm. Certain other dermatophytes develop only to a limited extent within the hair and their major development is around the outside of hair

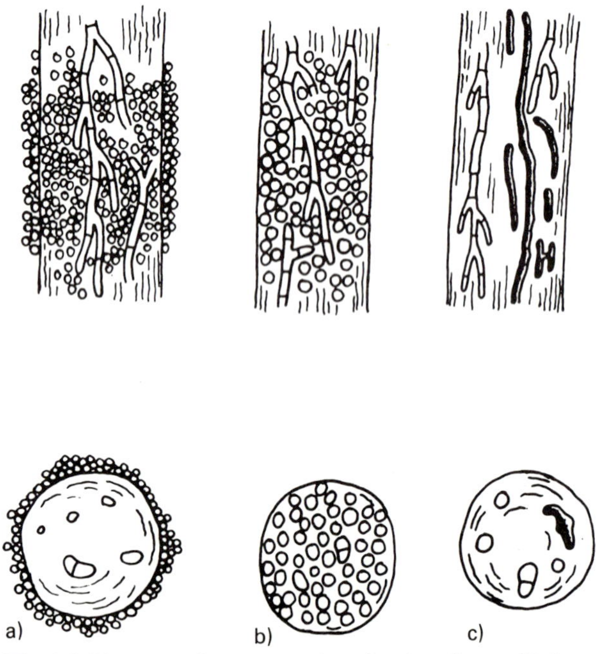

Fig. 6.5 Diagrammatic representation of various forms of hair invasion by dermatophytes as seen in longitudinal and transverse sections of hair shaft: (a) ectothrix (e.g. *M. audouinii*, *M. canis*, *T. mentagrophytes*) with hyphae sparsely distributed within hair shaft and a sheath of arthrospores on the outside; (b) endothrix (e.g. *T. tonsurans*, *T. violaceum*) with heavy arthrospore formation completely filling hair shaft; (c) favus (*T. schoenleinii*) showing sparse hyphal growth and formation of air spaces

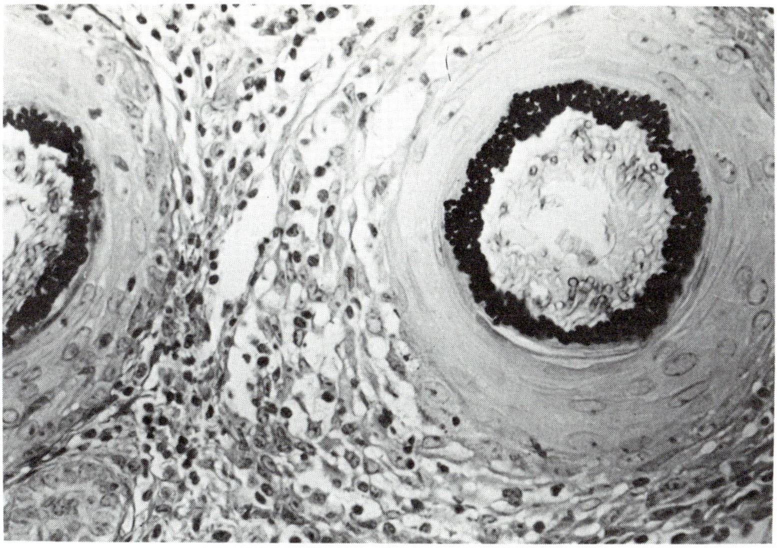

Fig. 6.6 Section of guinea pig skin infected with *Microsporum canis* and cut transversely through hair shafts showing sheath of arthrospores surrounding hairs. (× 450. Stained PAS)

shaft (ectothrix) where they produce a sheath of arthrospores (Fig. 6.6). In this type of hair invasion, characterized by *M. audouinii* infection, the hair usually breaks off about 2 mm above the mouth of the follicle. In the clinical condition called favus, caused by *T. schoenleinii*, the fungal activity within the hair shaft is minimal and the hair remains intact but intense fungal growth within and around the follicle produces the characteristic, waxy, honeycomb-like appearance on the scalp from which the name of the disease is derived.

Infections are often classified clinically as tinea capitis (scalp ringworm) or tinea pedis (foot ringworm) etc., according to the site affected, but these terms are for convenience only as they bear little or no relationship to the clinical appearance of the lesion or the species of fungus involved.

EPIDEMIOLOGY

Ringworm is the only truly contagious mycosis. The majority (approx. 80%) of dermatophytes do not occur as saprophytes in nature and are known only as agents of disease. Of these, about half are anthro-

Table 6.1 Common dermatophyte species: main host(s), site(s) of infection and distribution

Species	Common host(s), habitat, sites of infection*	Characteristics of hair infection †	Distribution	Remarks
Anthropophilic				
Epidermophyton floccosum	Groin, feet (nail)	–	Worldwide	Epidemics have been reported in institutions, gymnasia, etc.
Microsporum audouinii	Scalp (body)	S.S. ectothrix W.L. + ve	Common in Africa, America & Europe	Epidemics in children. Spontaneous cure at puberty
M. ferrugineum	Scalp (body)	S.S. ectothrix W.L. + ve	Africa, Balkans, Asia	Now rarely encountered
Trichophyton interdigitale	Feet (nail, groin)	–	Worldwide	Most common cause of foot ringworm in general population. Responds well to therapy
T. concentricum	Body	–	South Pacific	Causes bizarre pattern concentric lesions (Tinea imbricata)
T. rubrum	Feet, nail, groin, body	Rarely occurs	Worldwide	Most common cause of foot ringworm in clinic patients. Does not respond well to therapy
T. schoenleinii	Favus scalp (body, nail)	Endothrix with air spaces W.L. + ve (dull)	Common in Eurasia and N. Africa	Small pockets of infection in UK. Reservoir is longstanding subclinical infections — mainly in older females
T. soudanense	Scalp (body)	Endothrix	Common in Africa	Diagnosed occasionally in immigrants to UK
T. tonsurans	Scalp, body (nail)	Endothrix	Common in Europe and America	Black dot ringworm. Causes outbreaks in institutions. Reservoir in longstanding subclinical infections — mainly in older females
T. violaceum	Scalp, body (nail)	Endothrix	Common in Africa, Eurasia	Black dot ringworm. Diagnosed in immigrants to UK

Zoophilic				
Microsporum canis	Cat, dog	S.S. ectothrix W.L. + ve	Worldwide	Predominant cause of scalp ringworm in Britain and certain other temperate zones
M. distortum	Cat, dog	S.S. ectothrix	Australasia, USA	Rare. May be mutant form of *M. canis*
M. nanum	Pig	L.S. ectothrix	Worldwide	Rare. Also found in soil associated with pigs
M. persicolor	Bank/field voles	–	Europe	Rare
Trichophyton mentagrophytes	Rodents (horse, cat, dog)	S.S. ectothrix	Worldwide	A complex of species. Able to persist in soil for short periods of time
T. equinum	Horse	L.S. ectothrix	Worldwide	Epizootic in horses. Autotrophic var. Australia
T. erinacei	Hedgehog	–	Britain, N. Zealand	30% hedgehogs infected
T. quinckeanum	Mice	Favus	Europe, N. America	Infection commonly transferred to cats
T. simii	Monkey, chicken	–	India	Also found in soil
T. verrucosum	Cattle	L.S. ectothrix	Worldwide	Transfer to horse, dog, sheep common
Geophilic				
Microsporum fulvum	Soil	L.S. ectothrix W.L. + ve (rare, variable)	Worldwide	Sporadic infections, animals and man
M. gypseum	Soil	L.S. ectothrix W.L. + ve (rare, variable)	Worldwide	Sporadic infections, animals and man

† S.S. = Small spore ectothrix (arthrospores 2–5 μm diam.)
L.S. = Large spore ectothrix (arthrospores 5–8 μm diam.)
Endothrix (arthrospores 4–8 μm diam.)
W.L. = Wood's light.
* For zoophilic and geophilic species, infection in man occurs most commonly on exposed sites of the body and scalp.

pophiles, restricted to man as host; the others, the zoophiles, are primarily animal pathogens but also infect man. The few dermatophytes that occur naturally as saprophytes on keratinous material in soil (geophiles) cause occasional infection of both animals and man.

A number of saprophytic soil fungi are closely related to dermatophytes, sharing with them the ability to utilize keratin as a growth substrate and it is believed that the dermatophytes have evolved from these keratinophilic soil fungi. In the course of this evolutionary process various dermatophyte species have become adapted to particular hosts and this has eventually led to the development of the epidemiological groups of anthropophilic and zoophilic species. Similarly, within these groups further specialization has resulted in certain species being most frequently associated with a particular animal or a particular site of infection in man. Consequently, the anthropophilic dermatophytes can be subdivided into species which commonly cause infections of the scalp and body (e.g. *T. tonsurans*, *T. violaceum*) and those which most frequently occur as agents of foot, nail and groin ringworm (e.g. *T. rubrum*, *E. floccosum*). The zoophilic dermatophytes can likewise be associated with the particular species of animal which they most often infect, for example, *M. canis* with cats and dogs, *T. verrucosum* with cattle (Table 6.1).

Ringworm infection results from the transfer of arthrospores or keratinous material containing fungus from the infected to the uninfected. Frequently this transfer is indirect, for example, via the floors of shower stalls or by brushes, combs, towels, animal grooming implements and the like. Dermatophytes can remain viable for long periods of time within fomites and the interval between deposition and transfer may be considerable. In addition to exposure to the fungus, some abnormality of the epidermis, such as slight peeling or minor trauma, is probably necessary for the establishment of infection.

Records of ringworm go back as far as the 14th century and until some 50 years ago the most common form of the disease was ringworm of the scalp with associated infection of the body caused by anthropophilic dermatophytes. With improvements in living conditions, and in diagnosis, treatment and control of infection, the incidence of this form of ringworm has been considerably reduced and is now of significance only in certain Third World countries. In developed countries, ringworm of the scalp now accounts for only a small proportion of diagnosed infections and about 80% of these are caused by dermatophytes of animal origin. There is a significant reservoir of infection in the animal population and there is no evidence that this has increased nor been measurably reduced during recent times. However, the widespread and frequent use of communal bathing facilities in industry and in sporting and leisure establishments, has resulted in a very considerable increase in the incidence of foot ringworm and associated nail and groin infections caused by anthropophilic dermatophytes. These now comprise about three-quarters of all ringworm infections diagnosed in temperate zones.

There is no evidence of natural immunity to ringworm and although the young and the debilitated are apparently more susceptible to some forms of the disease, both sexes and all ages may become infected. Scalp ringworm is predominantly a disease of children and foot ringworm a disease of adults, particularly adult males.

PATHOGENESIS

Dermatophytes attack and degrade keratin in vitro by a combination of enzymatic digestion and mechanical pressure. In vivo, their activity is restricted to the zone of differentiating or newly differentiated keratin (Fig. 6.7) and for infection to persist the hyphal growth must keep pace with the rate of keratin production. Careful examination of the base of an infected hair for example, shows the actively growing hyphae poised for growth downwards into the differentiating keratin (Fig. 6.8), whilst in the mature keratin older hyphae and arthrospores are in the process of being carried upwards by the outgrowth of the hair. Similarly the fungal material present in the mature keratin of infected nails and horny layer of the skin is no longer involved in the disease process but invasion of new keratin continues. The desquamated horny layer, broken hairs and nail fragments

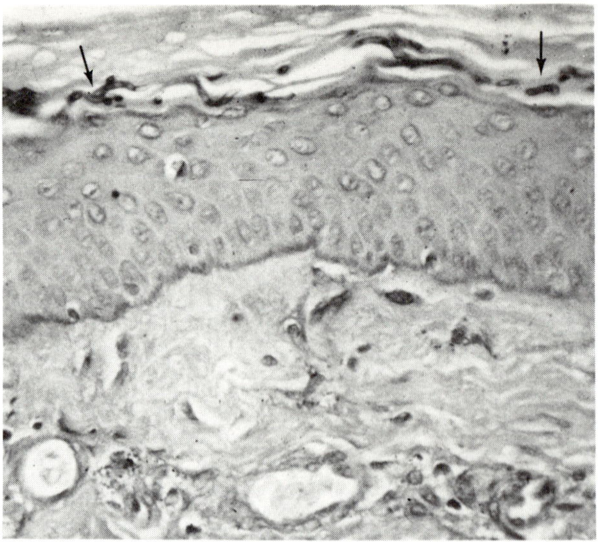

Fig. 6.7 Section of glabrous skin (*T. rubrum* infection) showing fungal hyphae confined to base of the horny layer (× 350. Stained PAS)

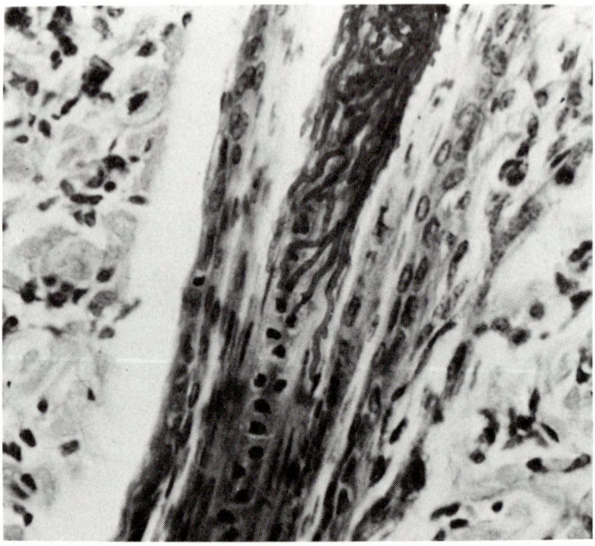

Fig. 6.8 Section of guinea pig skin infected with *Microsporum canis* cut longitudinally through hair shaft showing fungal hyphal growth restricted to zone of newly formed keratin (Adamson's fringe) (× 450. Stained PAS)

from infected sites do, however, contain viable fungus, sometimes in considerable amounts, and these form a source for the spread of infection.

The infective process ceases and cure occurs when the balance of fungus and host is disturbed in favour of the host and the upward movement of keratin carries the active dermatophyte hyphae away from the keratogenous zone.

MYCOLOGY

Dermatophytes are best considered for practical purposes as members of the Deuteromycotina although the perfect or sexual reproductive states of many of them are known. Three genera are recognized, namely, *Trichophyton*, *Microsporum* and *Epidermophyton*. This classification is based on the morphology of the macroconidia (Figs 6.9, 6.10) but dermatophytes are notoriously variable in their morphology and many isolates fail to produce these

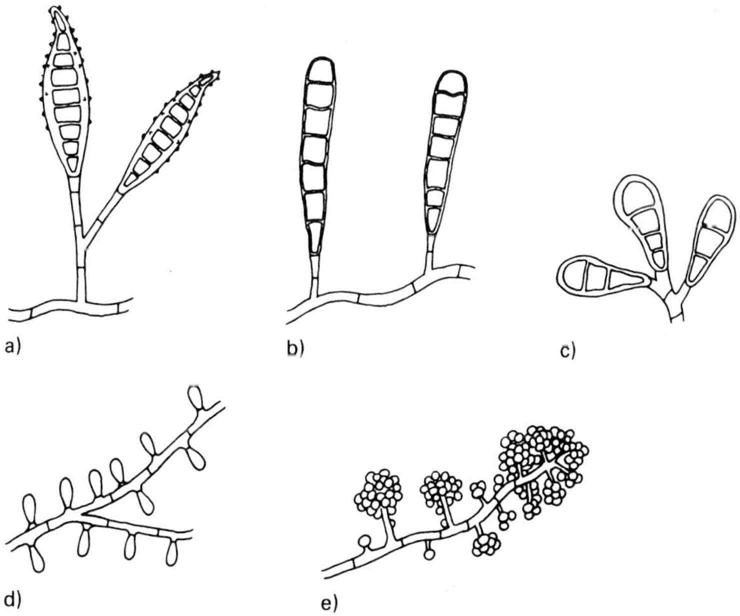

Fig. 6.9 Dermatophyte spore forms: (a) macroconidia of *Microsporum*; (b) macroconidia of *Trichophyton*; (c) macroconidia of *Epidermophyton*; (d) microconidia along sides of vegetative hyphae (en thyrses); (e) microconidia in grape-like bunches (en grappe)

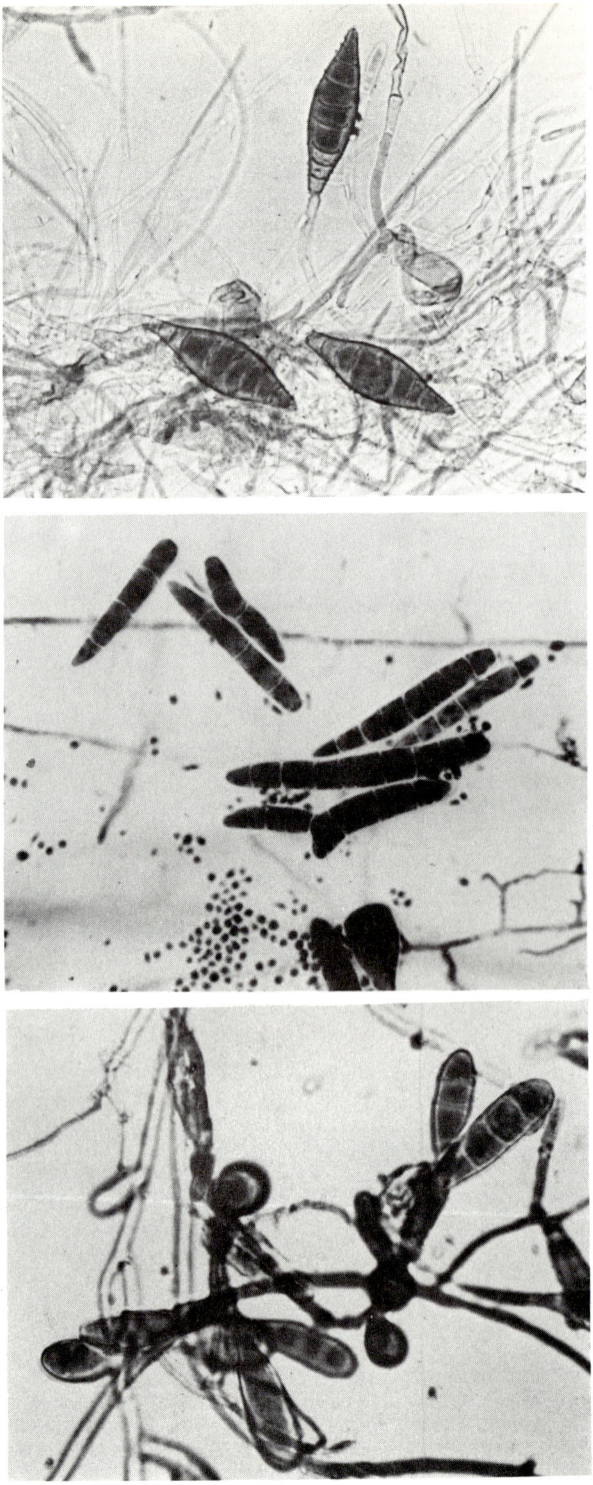

a)

b)

c)

Fig. 6.10 Macroconidia of dermatophytes; (a) *Microsporum canis*; (b) *Trichophyton rubrum*; (c) *Epidermophyton floccosum* (× 300. Cotton Blue/lactophenol) characteristic spores. The unicellular microconidia, their shape and disposition on the spore-bearing hyphae and other features such as spirals and racquet hyphae (Fig. 6.11) are therefore also used as features for identification, as are the macroscopic characteristics of the colony, such as texture, colour, growth rate and pigment production. For some species which produce little other than branched hyphae in culture, the form of the colony is paramount.

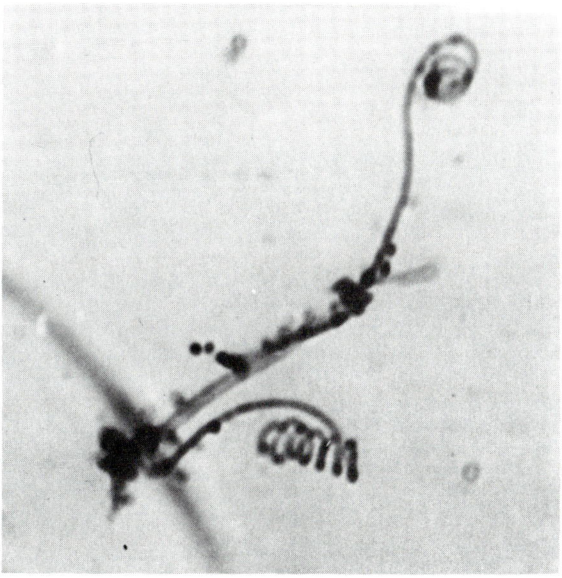

a)

Fig. 6.11 Vegetative structures formed by dermatophytes: (a) spiral hyphae; (b) racquet hyphae (× 380. Cotton Blue/lactophenol)

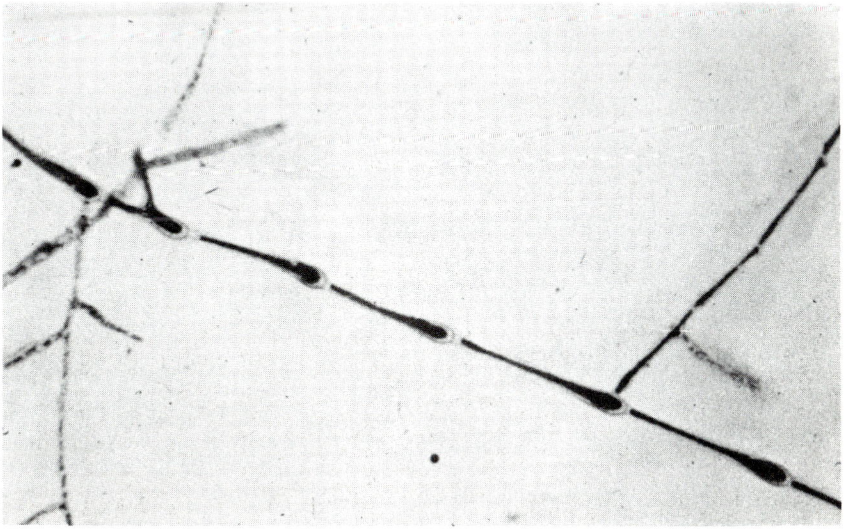

b)

Sexual reproduction

All dermatophytes for which the perfect state is known (Table 6.2) are heterothallic and both mating strains must be present for sexual reproduction to occur (Fig. 6.12). In addition, growth must take

Table 6.2 The perfect (sexual) states of dermatophytes

Imperfect state	Perfect state
Microsporum canis	*Nannizzia otae*
M. fulvum *	*N. fulva*
M. gypseum group	*N. gypsea* *N. incurvata*
M. nanum	*N. obtusa*
M. persicolor	*N. persicolor*
Trichophyton mentagrophytes group **	*Arthroderma benhamiae* *A. vanbreuseghemii*
T. simii	*A. simii*

* Although originally described as a separate species, *M. fulvum* was subsequently, and for many years until the perfect state was discovered, considered as a synonym of *M. gypseum*, and there are good reasons still for considering it to be a member of the *M. gypseum* group.

** Within the *T. mentagrophytes* group there are a number of recognizable 'strains' or varieties such as *T. interdigitale*, *T. erinacei*, *T. quinckeanum*, for which the relationships are uncertain and which are best retained for the present as separate species.

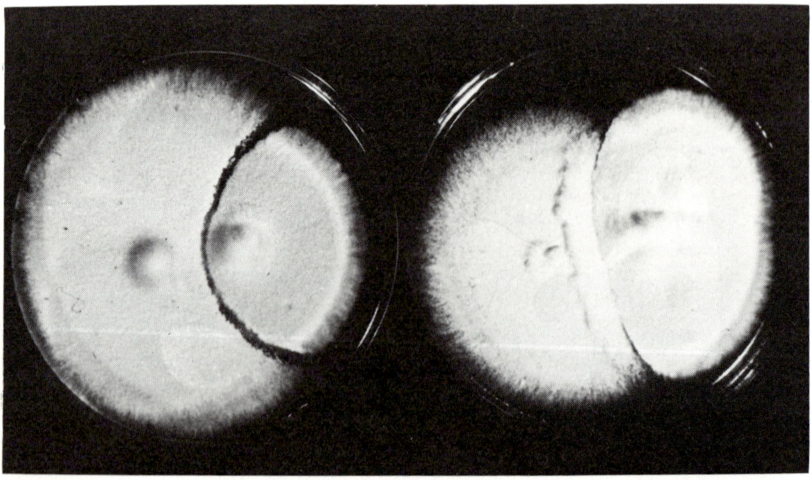

Fig. 6.12 Demonstration of heterothallism in keratinophilic fungi. Left hand petri-dish, cultures of the same mating strain of different species show zone of inhibition. On the right, different species of fungi but compatible (opposite) mating strains form a zone of stimulated growth

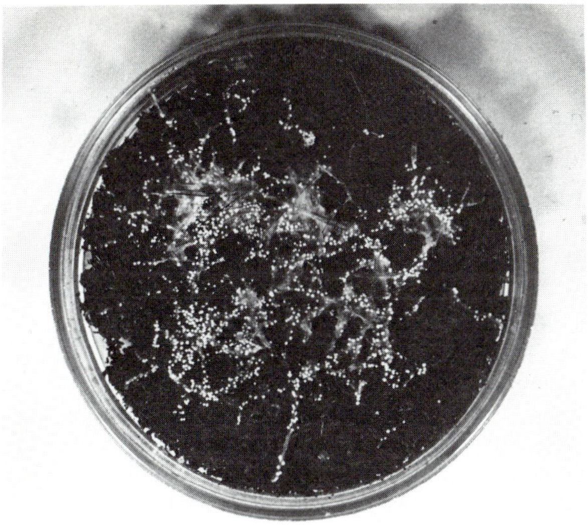

Fig. 6.13 Sexual reproduction of dermatophytes. Profuse formation of cleistothecia of *Nannizzia incurvata*, a perfect state of *Microsporum gypseum*, in soil/hair culture

place on a suitable substrate under conditions which simulate the natural habitat of geophilic species, such as is provided by either a complex carbohydrate or a keratin substrate within a hostile environment such as unsterile soil (Fig. 6.13). Sexual reproduction will not take place if an easily assimilated nutrient source is available.

All the known perfect states of the dermatophytes belong to the Ascomycotina in the order Eurotiales and family Gymnoascaceae. The cleistothecia (Fig. 6.14) are globose with a peridium (wall) composed of a basketwork of hyphae with thick-walled cells and for which the cell shape and/or hyphal branching is characteristic for the species. Within the peridium, large numbers of small asci, each containing eight lens-shaped ascospores are distributed irregularly.

The discovery of the perfect states and of the methods for their production in the laboratory has given us important new information about the ringworm fungi. It has been found, for example, that certain species such as *M. gypseum* and *T. mentagrophytes* have more than one perfect state and that these imperfect fungi therefore represent a complex of

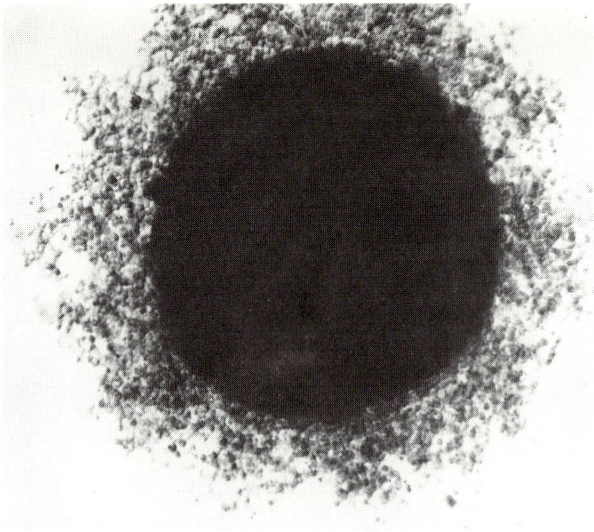

Fig. 6.14 Cleistothecium of dermatophyte showing wall (peridium) composed of ornately branched hyphae surrounding dense mass of asci and ascospores (× 75. Light Green/ lactophenol)

species which cannot easily be separated by study of their asexual and vegetative characteristics. It has also been found that some of the common dermatophytes, such as *T. rubrum* and *M. audounii*, apparently exist as single mating types indicating that their compatible mating strains may have been lost during evolution, perhaps because they were less well adapted to a parasitic existence.

DIAGNOSIS

Direct examination

Microscopical examination of KOH mounts of keratinous material is simple and reliable. The fungus is seen as a branching hyaline mycelium (Fig. 6.15) which frequently shows arthrospore production, particularly in infected hair (Fig. 6.16). However, in *T. schoenleinii* infection (favus) very little fungal growth takes place within the hair (Fig.6.17). With practice, artefacts can be easily differentiated from fungal structures. 'Mosaic fungus', for example, the most commonly encountered artefact in skin specimens, is distinguished from true fungus by its irregular outline and because it lies along the edges of the

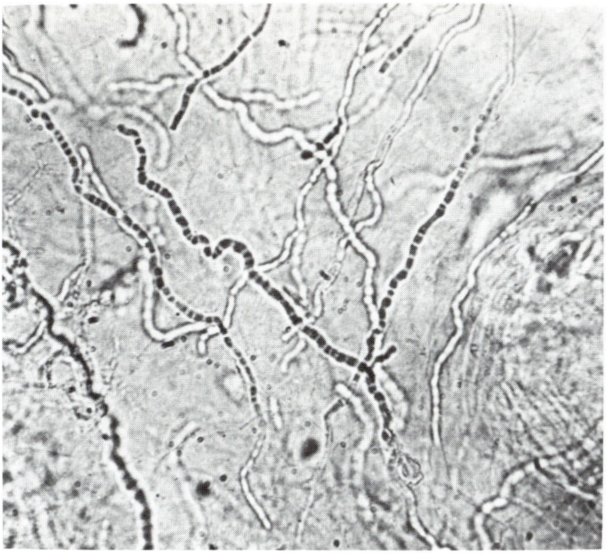

Fig. 6.15 KOH mount of dermatophyte infected skin scrapings showing branched hyphae and arthrospores (× 300)

cell walls, in contrast to fungal hyphae which are disposed quite independently of cell walls and frequently traverse their boundaries.

Microscopical examination should be made using a low intensity light source to ensure a good degree of contrast between the fungus and the keratinous substrate. Clearing of the specimen may be hastened by gentle warming of the mount but great care must be taken to avoid over-heating and crystallization of the KOH. The rate of clearing is enhanced if a mixture of KOH and DMSO (dimethyl-sulphoxide 40% v/v) is used but the degree of contrast between fungus and keratin is reduced in this mountant. Mounting in a KOH/Parker Quink ink mixture (50% v/v) can be helpful but it should be noted that artefacts as well as fungus are stained blue.

It is not possible to identify dermatophyte species by their morphology in skin and nail, although in hair infections the size and disposition of arthrospores can indicate which group of species is involved.

Culture

Dermatophytes develop well on culture media containing on organic source of nitrogen. Those

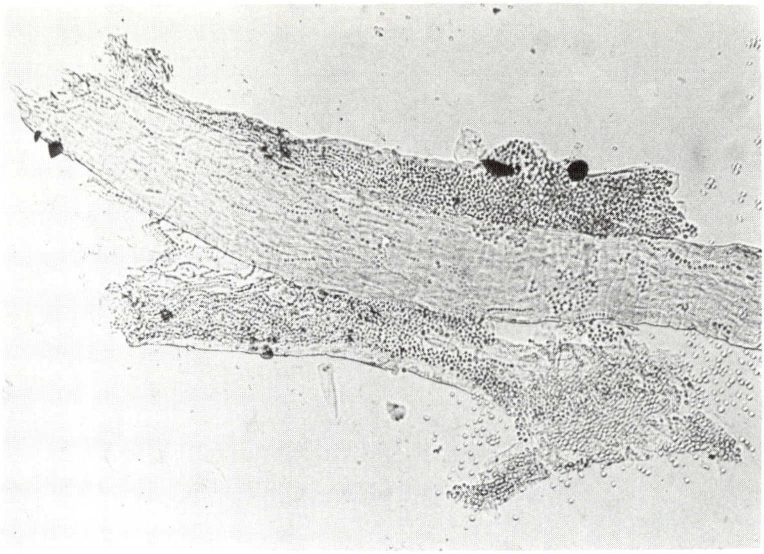

a)

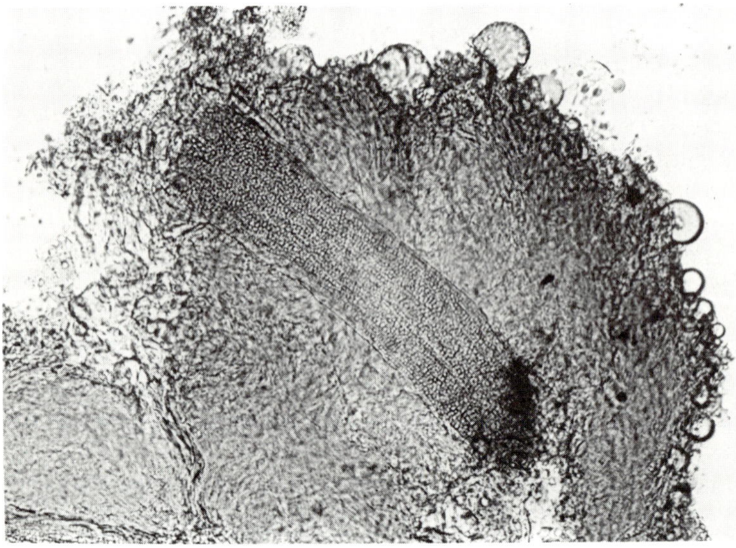

b)

Fig. 6.16 KOH mounts of dermatophyte infected hair (× 100): (a) ectothrix — the sheath of arthrospores has ruptured and lies adjacent to hair shaft; (b) endothrix with densely packed arthrospores within the hair shaft

commonly used for isolation are 4% malt extract and Sabouraud's dextrose agar and it is usual to supplement these media with chloramphenicol to reduce bacterial growth. If contamination with sapro-

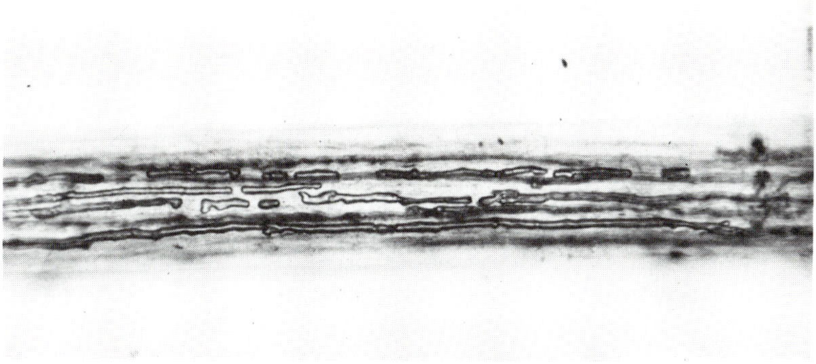

Fig. 6.17 Favus (*T. schoenleinii*) infected hair showing air spaces in hair shaft (× 100. KOH)

phytic fungi is likely to be troublesome, for example with specimens from nail or from animals, the medium may also be supplemented with cycloheximide (Actidione) which inhibits the development of most common fungal contaminants but to which the dermatophytes are highly resistant. Inoculation of an adequate number (⩾10) of small (<1 mm) fragments of the specimen should be made and although many dermatophytes may develop recognisable colonies within 5–7 days, cultures should be retained for at least 3 weeks at 25–30 °C and slightly longer at lower temperatures before discarding. At 37 °C the development of most dermatophytes is noticeably slower and this temperature is recommended only for the isolation of *T. verrucosum* which also develops better on a rich medium such as nutrient agar. Either petri dish or test-tube culture is satisfactory and there is little risk of laboratory infection. However, the use of petri-dishes is not convenient if a number of different isolation media and/or supplements are to be used, which is often advisable, for example, if *T. verrucosum* is suspected or if heavy contamination with other fungi is likely.

Dermatophyte isolates can usually be distinguished from contaminants by the occurrence of compact growth around the inocula and by the colour of the colony which for dermatophytes, unlike many of the common contaminants, is never green, blue or black. If, as sometimes happens, an isolate fails to produce spores, then subculturing on Czapek-Dox medium which supplies only inorganic nitrogen may be helpful — dermatophytes fail to grow on this medium while most common contaminants show good growth.

In addition to micromorphology and colonial appearance special tests exist for the differentiation of certain morphologically similar species of dermatophyte. For example, the ability of *T. mentagrophytes* to rapidly produce urease distinguishes it from *T. rubrum* and the ability to grow on rice grains separates *M. canis* from *M. audouinii*.

Wood's light

Hairs infected with *M. audouinii, M. Canis* and *T. schoenleinii* (Table 6.1) fluoresce under Wood's light, a source a long-wave ultraviolet light ('black light'). Wood's light may be used to assist clinical diagnosis and to select suitable material for laboratory investigation. In the laboratory it also enables selection of the best part of the hair for culture and direct examination. Care must be taken to differentiate between true fungal fluorescence (bright green) and the autofluorescence of keratin (dull blue) or the fluorescence of creams and ointments that may have been applied to the lesion.

Animal inoculation

Infections with a number of species can be established in guinea pigs but this is rarely a helpful or necessary diagnostic procedure.

Immunology and serology

The immunological aspects of ringworm are incompletely understood. It is clear that a primary infection produces partial local immunity to reinfection but this protection varies in duration and extent depending on the host, the site of infection and the species of dermatophyte. Cutaneous hypersensitivity (immediate and/or delayed) to dermatophyte skin test antigen (trichophytin) may occur and circulating antibodies have been detected in infected individuals but neither phenomenon has been shown to be of any diagnostic value.

Vesicular skin eruptions called 'id' reactions may occur, usually on the hand, in individuals with a ringworm infection particularly those with infections of the feet or scalp. They are believed to represent either hypersensitivity to circulating dermatophyte antigen, skin sensitizing antibodies or antigen/antibody complexes.

TREATMENT

Various topical preparations, for example, imidazole derivatives, Whitfield's ointment, tolnaftate or undecenoates. Oral griseofulvin, essential for nail and scalp infections. Some chronic infections require prolonged oral and topical therapy.

Chapter Seven SUPERFICIAL CANDIDOSIS

(Synonyms: superficial candidiasis; thrush)

Candidosis, a yeast infection caused by members of the genus *Candida*, occurs as a superficial disease involving the mucous membranes, skin or nails and also as a deep-seated infection which may be widely disseminated or be localized in one or more organ (Ch. 22). The causal fungi are common as commensals of many normal individuals and disease occurs only when there is some localized or general abnormality of the host. The superficial forms of candidosis are amongst the most frequently encountered infections in medical practice.

CLINICAL FORMS

Mucosal infections

Infections of the mouth and vagina are commonly referred to as thrush and are characterised by the development of discrete white patches on the mucosal surfaces which, if left untreated, may become confluent and form a curd-like pseudomembrane (Fig. 7.1).

Oral candidosis may affect any part of the buccal mucosa or the tongue and occurs most frequently in infancy and old age. Other forms occur in those who wear dentures, when lesions are restricted to the occluded area beneath the denture (denture stomatitis) and in some individuals antibiotic therapy may lead to the development of a painful *Candida* infec-

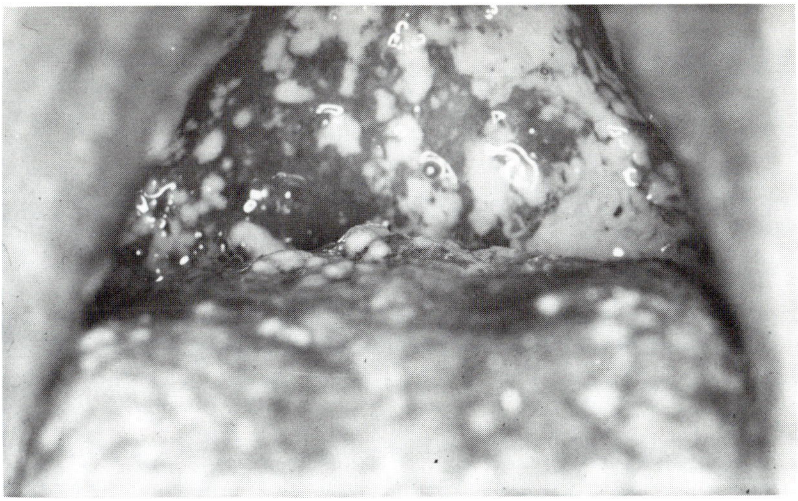

Fig. 7.1 Oral thrush caused by *Candida albicans*

tion of the tongue (antibiotic sore tongue). Infection of the lips with development of fissures at the angles of the mouth (angular cheilitis) is usually secondary to an infection of the mouth.

In vaginal thrush, typical white lesions occur on the epithelial surfaces of the vulva, vagina and cervix and are accompanied by itching and a milky-white discharge. Vaginal candidosis is common, particularly during pregnancy.

Skin and nail infections

Candida infection of the skin usually occurs on the sites that may become abnormally moist such as the axillae, groins, perineum, submammary folds and occasionally the toe-clefts. In infants, candidosis is important as a frequent complication of napkin dermatitis. Typically in skin infection there is scaling, maceration, acute inflammation and 'satellite lesions' peripheral to the main area of involvement.

Infection of the hands (usually the finger webs), the nail folds (paronychia) and nails (onychia) is associated with frequent immersion of the hands in water and is an occupational disease, for example among housewives and barmaids. The appearance of infected nails varies considerably but generally they become discoloured and there is erosion of the nail plate; the nail fold and the surrounding skin may or

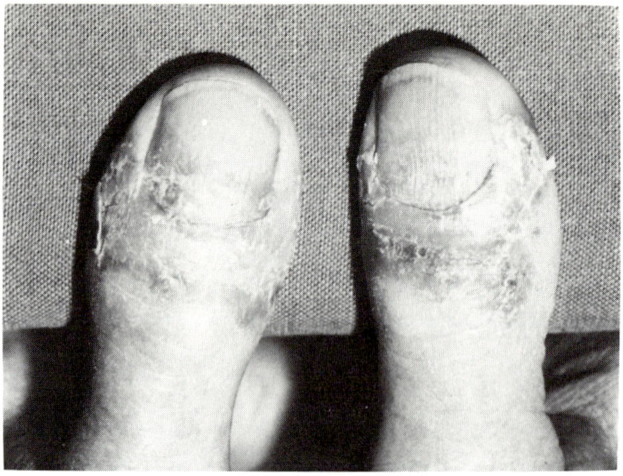

Fig. 7.2 Candidosis of nails and surrounding skin of fingers

may not be involved (Fig. 7.2). Paronychia is usually a chronic condition and is notoriously difficult to eradicate. It is caused by a mixed *Candida* and bacterial infection and characteristically there is pronounced swelling at the base of the nail with an associated accumulation of pus.

Superficial infections due to *Candida* also occur at other sites such as the penis (balanitis), often following sexual contact with females with vaginal candidosis, and the yeast may also infect the outer ear (otitis externa) (Ch. 10).

Chronic mucocutaneous candidosis (CMC)

This rare form of the disease which usually becomes apparent in childhood is a chronic, sometimes granulomatous infection of the mucosa, skin and nails. Those who develop CMC generally have underlying genetic abnormalities or endocrine disorders which result in defects in cellular immunity, usually in T-cell function, the magnitude of which determines the severity and extent of the lesions.

EPIDEMIOLOGY

Only rarely do pathogenic *Candida* species occur in the environment and then only in sites closely associated with man or animals, such as fomites in the hospital environment and soil containing recently deposited animal or bird droppings. These are only very occasional sources of infection and with the exception of sexually transmitted candidosis, the disease is considered to be one of endogenous origin.

Candida, in particular *C. albicans*, is present as a commensal of the mouth, intestinal tract and vagina of a considerable proportion of the normal population. The carriage rate tends to increase with age and is higher in the vagina during pregnancy.

Commensal yeasts are also more prevalent during illness and consequently they are widely distributed among hospitalized patients (Ch. 22).

A wide variety of factors are known to predispose to both superficial and deep *Candida* infection and the most important of these are summarized in Table 7.1. All act either by altering the balance of the normal microbial flora of the body or by lowering resistance to infection. Some exert specific or local effects whereas others have a more generalized influence. Infection is most likely when several factors operate together to compound these effects.

Table 7.1 Factors that predispose to yeast overgrowth and *Candida* infection

Pathological/physiological
Natural receptive states, e.g. infancy, pregnancy, old age
Severe or chronic underlying infection
Endocrine disorders, e.g. diabetes mellitus, hypoparathyroidism
Defects in cell-mediated immunity
Malignancies (carcinoma and leukaemia)
Drug addition — accidental bloodstream inoculation
Mechanical
Trauma — including burns
Local occlusion and maceration of tissues
Iatrogenic
Drug therapy — altering endogenous flora or suppressing local immunity, e.g. antibiotics, oral contraceptives, corticosteroids, cytotoxic and immunosuppressive agents
Surgical procedures, e.g. heart, gastrointestinal, brain and transplantation surgery
Intravenous catheters — contamination and accidental bloodstream inoculation

MYCOLOGY

The genus *Candida* comprises more than 100 species of asporogenous yeasts classified within the Deuteromycotina including species which were until recently classified in the genus *Torulopsis*. Eight species are firmly established as pathogens and all are found predominantly in close association with man or warm-blooded animals. The most frequently encountered and most virulent is *C. albicans* while the others in descending order of virulence are *C. tropicalis*, *C.* (*Torulopsis*) *glabrata*, *C. parapsilosis*, *C. pseudotropicalis*, *C. krusei*, *C. guilliermondii* and *C. viswanathii*. The pathogenic status of the few other *Candida* species which have been reported to cause disease is doubtful.

Although *C. albicans* accounts for 80–90% of infections overall, there is a frequent association between certain other species and particular forms of the disease. For example, *C. glabrata* is common in vaginal infections whilst infections of nails due to *C. parapsilosis* and *C. guilliermondii* outnumber those caused by *C. albicans*.

The pathogenic species grow predominantly in the yeast phase as round–oval cells (3–8 μm diam.) on common media such as Sabouraud's dextrose agar and as a mixture of yeast cells, pseudomycelium and true mycelium in vivo or under special cultural conditions. *C. glabrata* is an exception in that it never forms mycelium or pseudomycelium.

DIAGNOSIS

Clinically, superficial forms of candidosis can be confused with other diseases. However, laboratory diagnosis is relatively straightforward.

Direct examination

In scrapings from lesions of the skin, nails or mucous membranes examined microscopically in KOH, the fungus may be seen as budding yeast cells and in the majority of instances mycelium is also present (Fig. 7.3); the relative quantity of the two growth

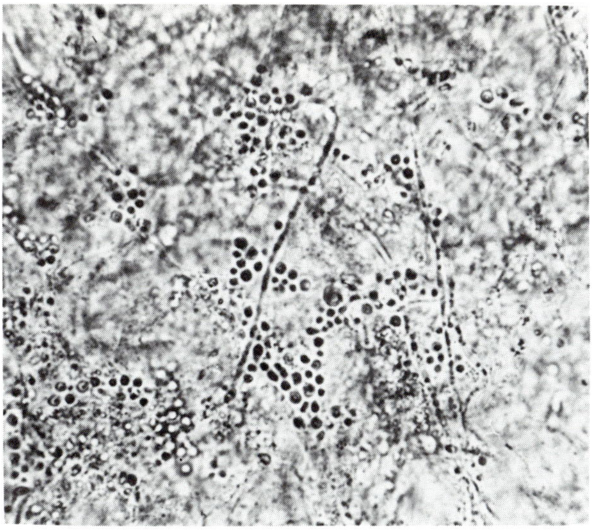

Fig. 7.3 Skin scrapings showing yeast cells and hyphae of *Candida albicans* (× 100. KOH)

phases varies considerably and in the case of *C. glabrata* infections mycelium is absent.

Culture

Candida species grow well in culture on common isolation media such as Sabouraud's dextrose agar at 25–37 °C and typical yeast colonies usually develop within 24 hours. Isolates can be identified by the standard fermentation and assimilation tests or by using one of the commercial kits for identification of medically important yeasts which are now available. However, since *C. albicans* accounts for the majority of isolates it is usual for the simpler tests of germ tube formation or chlamydospore production to be used first of all for identification of this species (Fig. 7.4).

In suspected superficial candidosis, confirmation by microscopy that yeasts and mycelium are present in material from lesions together with isolation of the yeast in culture is sufficient for diagnosis.

Animal inoculation

This procedure is of no value for determining the significance or the identification of *Candida* isolates.

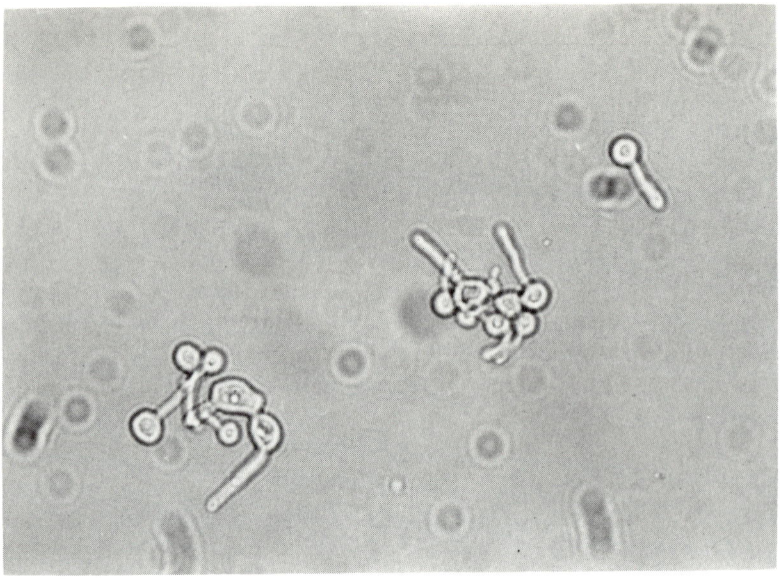

a)

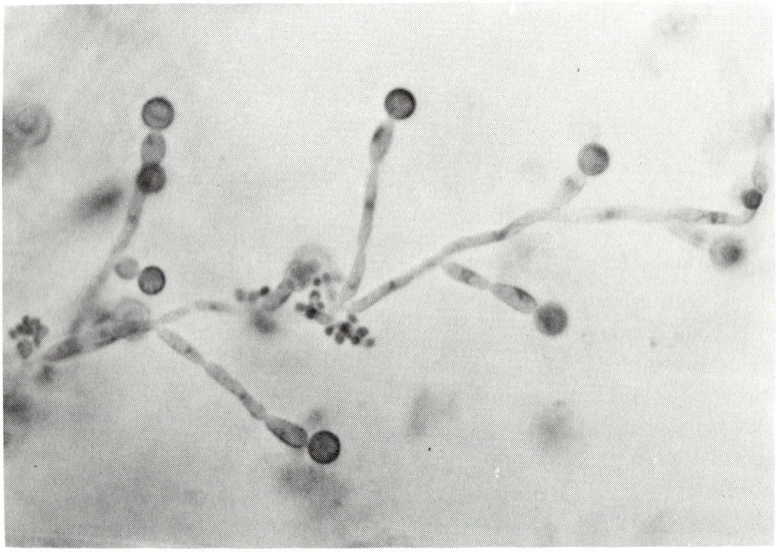

b)

Fig. 7.4 Rapid identification of *Candida albicans*: (a) germ tubes formed in serum after $1\frac{1}{2}$ h at 37°C (× 360); (b) chlamydospore formation on Czapek Dox + Tween 80 agar (× 200)

Immunology and serology

Skin tests

These are of no diagnostic value for candidosis as the majority of the population give a positive reaction.

Serological tests

These are neither useful nor necessary for diagnosis of superficial candidosis.

TREATMENT

Topical nystatin, amphotericin B or imidazole derivatives. Keeping site of infection dry will have significant beneficial effect. Oral ketoconazole for intractable chronic infections including chronic mucocutaneous candidosis for which immunological reconstitution may also be required.

Chapter Eight PITYRIASIS VERSICOLOR

(Synonym: tinea versicolor)

Pityriasis versicolor, caused by the lipophilic yeast *Malassezia furfur*, is a mild, chronic infection of the stratum corneum which, as the name indicates, causes a patchy discolouration of the skin.

CLINICAL FORMS

The trunk, upper limbs, neck and face are the most commonly affected areas but any part of the body may be involved. Lesions are usually numerous, well demarcated and non-inflammatory with only fine scaling. The fungus interferes with melanin production and the lesions vary in appearance according to the degree of pigmentation of the surrounding skin. In dark-skinned races or on areas of tanned skin, the lesions are always lighter in colour than the adjacent normal skin. In light-skinned individuals lesions appear as pale brown, hyperpigmented patches (Fig. 8.1) and these are often hardly noticeable until exposure to sunlight renders them more obvious by their failure to tan.

The fungus is located mainly in the upper layers of the stratum corneum (Fig. 8.2) and the major effect of the disease is cosmetic; only occasionally is there a host response such as mild inflammation or pruritus.

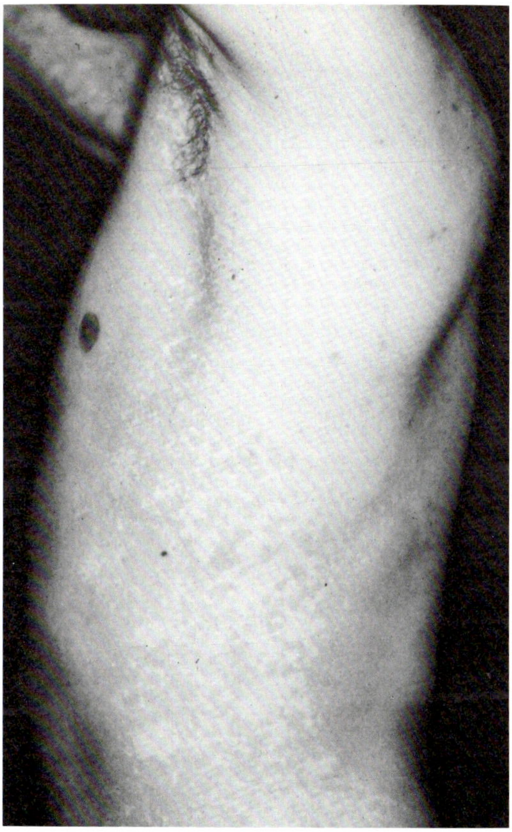

Fig. 8.1 Pityriasis versicolor in young adult male showing hyperpigmented lesions on the trunk

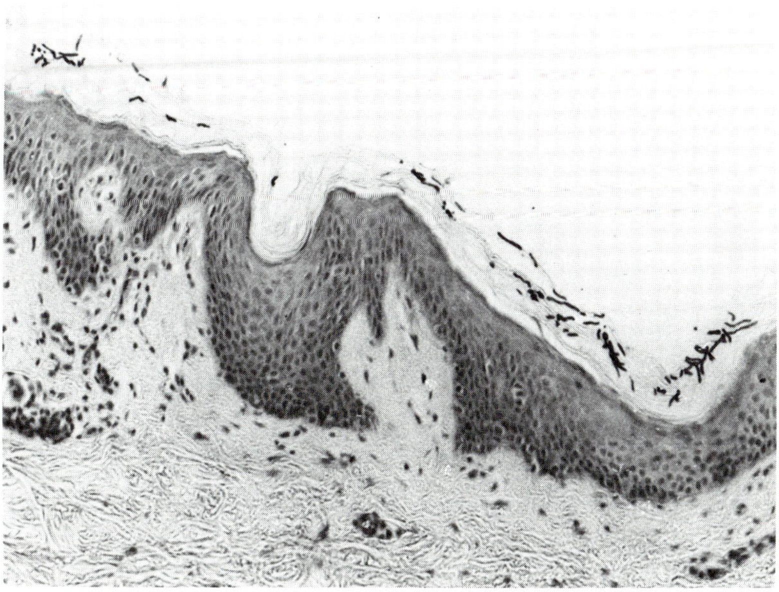

Fig. 8.2 Biopsy section showing the hyphae and yeast cells of *Malassezia furfur* concentrated mainly in the upper layers of the stratum corneum; compare with Fig. 6.7 (× 100. Stained PAS)

EPIDEMIOLOGY

The causal fungus *Malassezia furfur* is a member of the normal microflora of the skin of many individuals and contagious spread of the disease, although it occasionally occurs, is not thought to play a significant role in its epidemiology. Consequently, the conditions which lead to the development of the disease, although not precisely known, are most likely to be related to host or environmental factors. There is a much higher incidence of infection in warm climates than in temperate zones and also in individuals with illnesses causing high temperature or necessitating long periods confined to bed, indicating that excessive sweating is probably one of the predisposing factors.

The disease occurs in all age groups but is apparently most prevalent in young adults. No differences in the incidence of infection according to sex or race have been noted.

MYCOLOGY

Attempts to isolate the causal fungus in pure culture were unsuccessful for many years and it was described and named by study of its morphology in skin scales. When it was eventually isolated, by supplying its growth requirement for free fat, *M. furfur* was found to occur on the normal skin of both uninfected and infected individuals, as well as in disease lesions. In culture it develops as a yeast closely resembling *Pityrosporum ovale* (the bottle bacillus), an organism well known because of its association with dandruff scales. Because of its predominantly globose cells the isolate from pityriasis versicolor was named *Pityrosporum orbiculare*. It is now accepted, by most authorities, that *P. ovale* and *P. orbiculare* are conspecific and since the generic name *Malassezia* antedates that of *Pityrosporum*, the correct name for this fungus, according to the rules of nomenclature, is *M. furfur*.

DIAGNOSIS

Direct examination

The diagnosis is most conveniently and accurately made by microscopical examination of skin scales mounted in KOH. The fungus is usually present in quantity and the clusters of round yeast cells (5–8 μm diam.) together with short, stout hyphae which may be curved and occasionally branched, are easily recognized and very characteristic (Fig. 8.3).

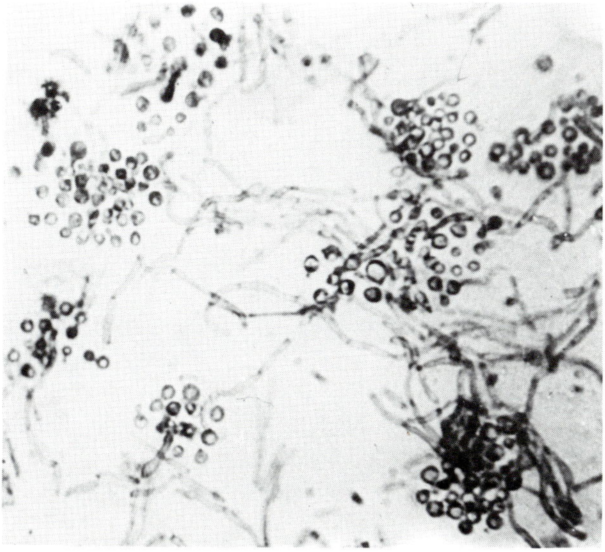

Fig. 8.3 Skin scrapings showing characteristic hyphae and clusters of yeast cells of *Malassezia furfur* (× 320. KOH)

Culture

Although seldom necessary for diagnostic purposes, the isolation of *M. furfur* in culture is easily achieved by inoculation of scrapings from the infected area on Sabouraud's dextrose agar overlayed with a film of olive oil. The small, creamy-yellow colonies develop within 5–7 days at 30 °C. Microscopical examination shows them to be composed of budding yeast cells, the majority of which are globose and 3–5 μm diameter (orbiculare type) with a number of small

(1–2.5 μm diam.) bottle-shaped cells (ovale type) also present. Hyphae are only occasionally produced in culture, usually as germ tubes from orbiculare-type cells.

TREATMENT

Topical 1% selenium sulphide, Whitfield's ointment or imidazole.

Chapter Nine OTHER SUPERFICIAL INFECTIONS OF SKIN, NAIL AND HAIR

SKIN AND NAIL

It is not unusual to isolate fungi other than dermatophytes or *Candida* species from abnormal skin and nails. In the majority of instances these are merely casual, transient contaminants and direct microscopical examination is usually either negative or if positive shows only very restricted and abnormal hyphal growth. However, certain non-dermatophytes are capable of causing infection and when this is so it is important that their significance is recognized since they are likely to be resistant to the agents used for the treatment of ringworm or candidosis.

Hendersonula toruloidea

Although usually diagnosed in temperate zones, infections with *Hendersonula toruloidea* are almost entirely restricted to individuals who are natives, or have been long-term residents of countries with tropical or subtropical climates. In Britain 20–30% of coloured immigrants with clinical symptoms of foot ringworm are infected with this fungus. The feet and toe-nails are most often affected, although infections of hands and finger-nails also occur and infection of the glabrous skin of the face and body has been reported on at least one occasion. Since first recognized in Britain, *H. toruloidea* infections have been reported from many parts of the world.

Clinical forms

Skin infections with *H. toruloidea* are clinically indistinguishable from ringworm but nail infections differ in that the nail usually becomes dark in colour and is generally less friable than a dermatophyte-infected nail. As with foot ringworm, *H. toruloidea* infection centres on the lateral toe-cleft and spreads from there to other parts of the foot, to the nails and to the hands. The fungus is resistant to the available topical antifungals and to griseofulvin.

Epidemiology

H. toruloidea is a common pathogen of fruit trees in many tropical and subtropical zones and it is presumed that infection is contracted as a result of contact with the fungus in soil by those who habitually go barefoot in these regions. Overt disease develops following the regular wearing of shoes and socks in those who emigrate to colder climates. There is no evidence to suggest that the disease is contagious or that spread of infection occurs in communal bathing places as it does for foot ringworm.

In Britain, infections have been diagnosed mainly in immigrants from the Indian subcontinent and West Africa.

Mycology

H. toruloidea is a member of the Sphaeropsidales, a group of pycnidial forming fungi within the Deuteromycotina. However, pycnidia are usually produced only after long periods (six weeks or more) of incubation in daylight on complex natural media. In most instances, isolates from man can be identified on the basis of the consistent isolation of grey-black colonies which on microscopical examination show coiled, hyaline hyphae and chains of dark coloured, thick-walled thallospores (Fig. 9.1).

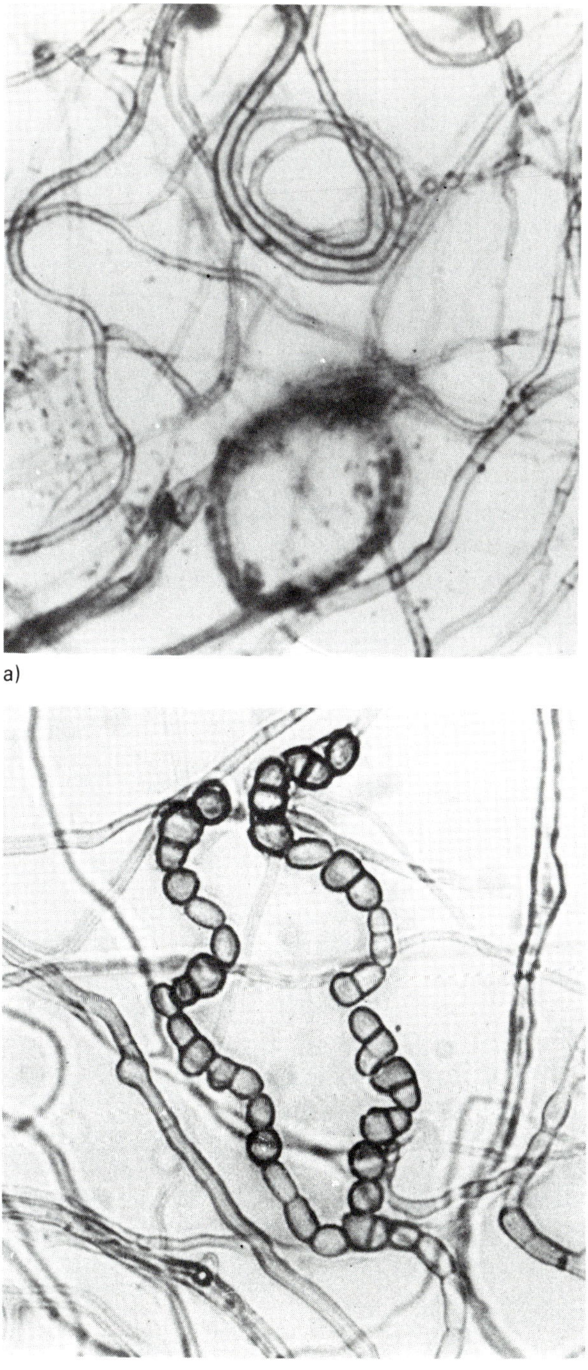

a)

b)

Fig. 9.1 Culture mounts of *Hendersonula toruloidea* showing (a) coiled, hyaline hyphae and (b) chains of dematiaceous, thick-walled thallospores (× 360. Lactophenol)

Diagnosis

Direct examination. KOH mounts of infected skin show hyaline, branched hyphae which cannot with certainly be differentiated from a dermatophyte, although arthrospores are not formed (Fig. 9.2). Dematiaceous, thick-walled thallospores may be present in nail.

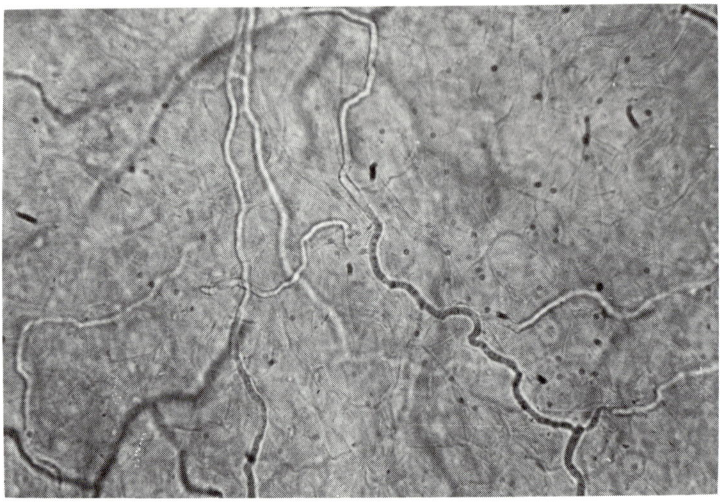

Fig. 9.2 Skin scrapings showing branched, spreading hyphae of *Hendersonula toruloidea*; arthrospores are not formed (× 300. KOH)

Culture. H. toruloidea is extremely sensitive to cycloheximide (Actidione) and this antibiotic must be omitted from at least some of the isolation media when attempting to culture specimens from suspected ringworm in individuals who come from a warm climate. Because it was customary in many laboratories to supplement all isolation media with cycloheximide it is certain that, prior to the discovery of *H. toruloidea* as a pathogen of man, many infections with this fungus were misdiagnosed as ringworm for which culture had failed.

Animal inoculation. Skin infection has been induced experimentally in laboratory animals (rabbits) but only with difficulty and animal inoculation is of no value for the purposes of identification of the fungus or the diagnosis of disease in man.

Scytalidium hyalinum

Since the recognition of *H. toruloidea* as a cause of skin and nail infections, the use of cycloheximide as a supplement in all isolation media was discontinued in many laboratores. In regions of Britain with a high proportion of immigrants from tropical and subtropical areas a second non-dermatophyte, *Scytalidium hyalinum*, was soon recognized as a cause of similar superficial infection. *S. hyalinum* differs from *H. toruloidea* mainly in being hyaline at all stages of growth. Like *H. toruloidea* it is very sensitive to cycloheximide and resistant to griseofulvin. All the individuals found to be infected have been immigrants from the West Indies or West Africa and it is presumed that, as for *H. toruloidea*, infection is contracted by contact with soil containing the fungus and that clinical symptoms develop as a result of occlusion of the feet by regular wearing of footwear.

Scopulariopsis brevicaulis

Scopulariopsis brevicaulis is as an ubiquitous saprophyte in soil and many other natural substrates worldwide. It is the most common cause of nail infection by a non-dermatophyte. Most frequently the great toe nail is involved and usually after damage by trauma or by infection with another organism such as a dermatophyte. As such, *Scopulariopsis* may be considered a secondary invader but once established it continues to develop and destroy the nail keratin. Since it is resistant to the therapeutic agents at present employed for treatment of dermatophyte infections it is important to differentiate between its occurrence as a contaminant and as an invader. This is best achieved by direct examination which usually reveals the presence of the characteristically roughened, bell-shaped, asexual conidia within the nail (Fig. 9.3). The number of colonies isolated in culture, and whether or not they originate from the inocula, can also be helpful in establishing the significance of isolates. Infections of skin with *S. brevicaulis* have also been documented but the validity of these reports is rather doubtful.

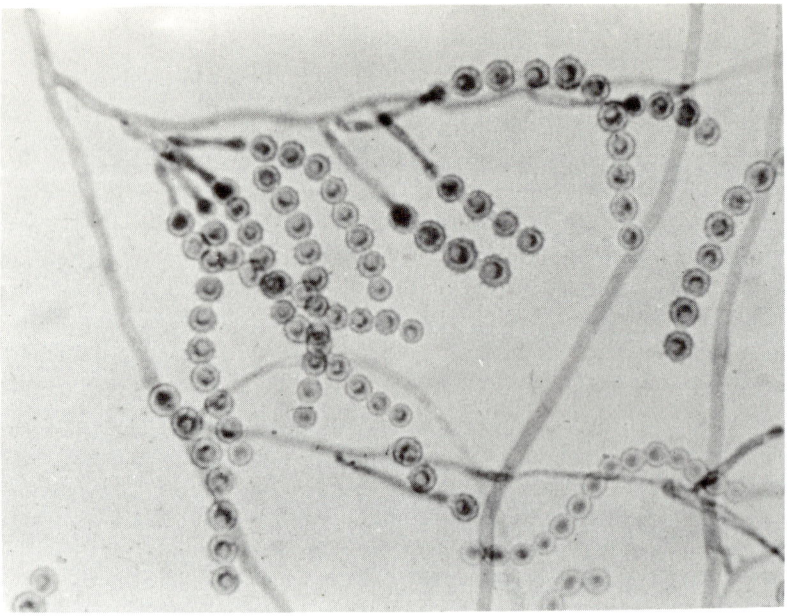

a)

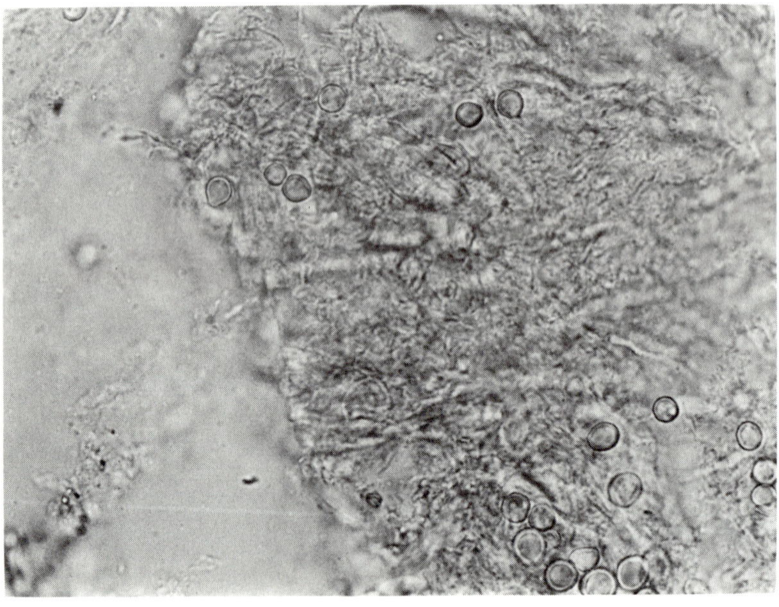

b)

Fig. 9.3 (a) Culture mount of *Scopulariopsis brevicaulis* showing roughened, bell-shaped spores (lactophenol); (b) Characteristic spores of *S. brevicaulis* in infected nail (KOH) (× 380)

Other fungi

Various common saprophytic fungi, such as *Fusarium*, *Aspergillus* and *Penicillium* species are occasionally implicated in nail infections, usually as secondary invaders following trauma. If isolated, the significance of these fungi can usually be established by microscopy of the nail, by the number of inocula which produce colonies and by repeated isolation from successive specimens.

Treatment

H. toruloidea, *S. hyalinum* and *S. brevicaulis* infections do not respond to the available topical or oral antifungals. Nails may be removed surgically but infection may recur.

Tinea nigra (*Exophiala (Cladosporium) werneckii*)

Tinea nigra is a superficial, asymptomatic skin disease characterized by brown to black areas of variable size usually affecting thickly keratinized regions such as the palms of the hands and the soles of the feet. It is considered to be a tropical disease and occurs commonly in Africa, Asia and Central and South America but is now being diagnosed more frequently in Europe and North America in immigrants and visitors returning from these regions. The causal fungus, *E. werneckii*, is confined to the outer layers of the stratum corneum where it grows profusely as densely packed and frequently branched, septate, dark-brown hyphae (Fig. 9.4). There is little tissue reaction or discomfort to the individual but there is a gradual peripheral spread of the darkly pigmented lesion. The disease differs fundamentally from ringworm in the lack of scaling, the colouration of the affected area and the restriction of fungal activity to the outer zone of the horny layer. Furthermore, the disease is not contagious and infection is contracted following contact with the causal fungus in soil. Diagnosis is easily made by recognition of the dematiaceous hyphae on microscopical examination of skin scrapings in KOH. Material may also be cultured at 25–30 °C on Sabouraud's dextrose agar and the fungus develops as light to dark grey yeast-

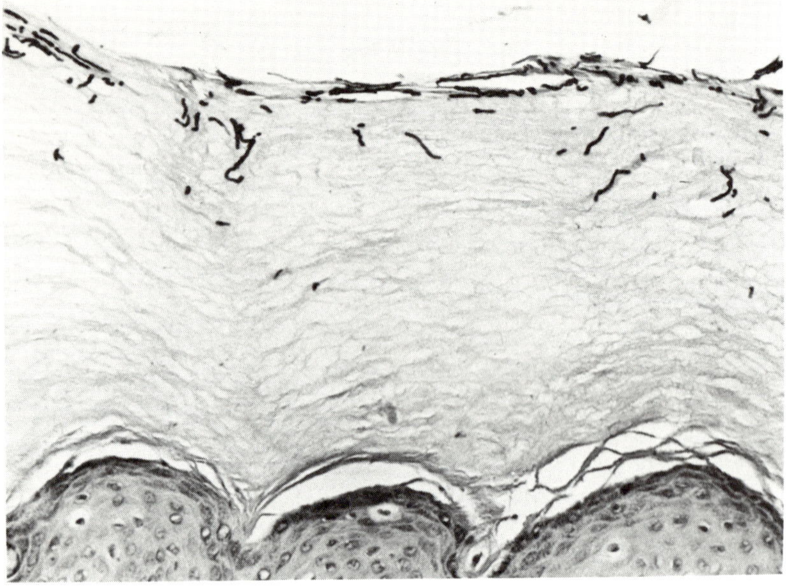

Fig. 9.4 Biopsy section of *Tinea nigra* showing the hyphae of *Exophiala werneckii* concentrated in the upper layers of the thick horny layer of the foot (× 300. Stained PAS)

like colonies becoming mycelial and dark olivaceous green to black with age.

The response to treatment with keratolytic agents is good. However, tinea nigra is important because outside of the regions where it commonly occurs, it may be misdiagnosed for the much more serious condition malignant melanoma which, clinically, it closely resembles.

HAIR

White piedra (*Trichosporon beigelii*)

This disease, which is characterized by soft white, greyish or light brown nodules on the hair shafts occurs mainly on the hair of the axillae. Because growth of the fungus within the hair may cause it to break at the point of infection a clubbed or swollen end to some of the hairs is common. *T. beigelii* is present as branched hyphae and arthrospores both within and around the hair. When cultured, moist yeast-like colonies containing blastospores, mycelium and arthrospores develop rapidly, changing from cream to yellowish-grey and becoming wrinkled and radially furrowed with age.

Shaving of the affected area is usually sufficient to effect a cure.

Black piedra (*Piedraia hortae*)

This disease is characterized by the presence on hairs of black, hard nodules up to 1 mm in diameter. Hairs of the beard and scalp may be affected and the disease is also found in primates. Black piedra occurs in countries with humid, tropical climates where the causal fungus is believed to live in the soil. Diagnosis is a relatively simple matter. Crushing the brittle nodules reveals locules containing club-shaped asci, and within each ascus are eight fusiform ascospores with a single, polar, spirally curved filament. Culture is not necessary for diagnosis of the disease but *P. hortae* will grow on agar media and although growth is slow and restricted, it will in time produce asci and ascospores.

Shaving to remove the affected hairs is a satisfactory form of treatment.

Chapter Ten FUNGAL INFECTIONS OF THE EYE AND EAR

MYCOTIC KERATITIS

(Synonym: keratomycosis)

Mycotic keratitis results from infection of the cornea of the eye, usually following injury, with fungi which occur commonly as saprophytes in nature. The incidence of this disease has increased as a result of the frequent use of antibacterial antibiotics and corticosteroids to treat eye conditions.

Clinical forms

The appearance of the disease is broadly similar irrespective of the species of fungus involved and is characterized by the presence on the cornea of a fluffy, white area, usually with an irregular border. This is accompanied by a severe inflammatory reaction and development of hypopyon (Fig. 10.1). However, clinical diagnosis in the early stages is difficult particularly if symptoms such as inflammation are masked by corticosteroid treatment.

Epidemiology

In most cases there is a history of trauma caused by vegetation or soil dust in which the causal fungi are commonly present in quantity. There is also, frequently, a history of treatment with antibacterial antibiotics and/or corticosteroids. The wide range of fungi reported as causal agents and the association of infection with the use of agents which influence host

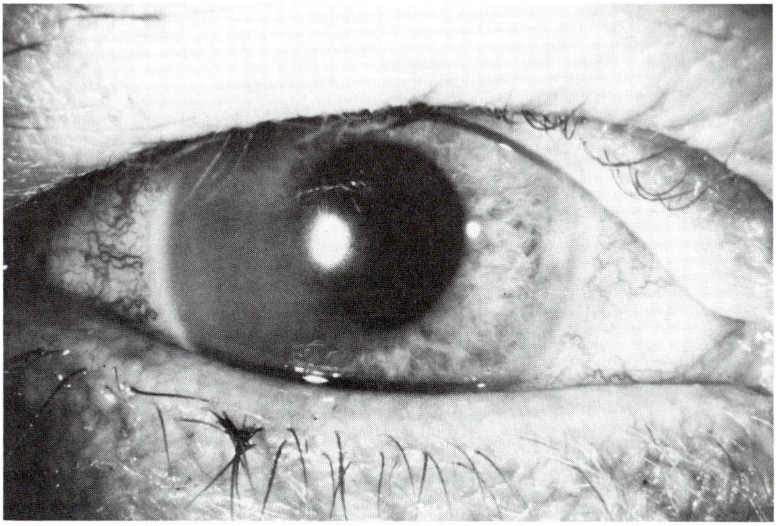

Fig. 10.1 Mycotic keratitis due to *Fusarium solani* showing abscess formation and hypopyon (photograph courtesy of Mr B. Noble, General Infirmary, Leeds)

resistance emphasizes the opportunistic nature of the disease. Mycotic keratitis has a worldwide distribution but occurs more frequently in warm, dry climates than in temperate zones and it is more common among agricultural workers than in any other occupation.

Mycology

Many different fungi have been reported as the cause of mycotic keratitis but as many of these species have also been isolated from healthy eyes and are also commonly encountered as laboratory contaminants, doubt exists about the authenticity of some reports. Nevetherless, species of *Aspergillus* and *Fusarium* are confirmed as the most common causal fungi.

Diagnosis

Since the fungi involved are opportunistic pathogens, culture alone is insufficient for diagnosis and the major effort should be aimed at finding fungal elements by direct examination. This does not allow the species to be determined but in any case this will seldom affect treatment.

Direct examination

Superficial swabs are of little value and corneal scrapings should be taken. The fungal elements may be rather sparse and difficult to find and, although KOH mounts may be satisfactory, it is advisable to stain a representative portion of the material with the PAS or methenamine-silver techniques; the fungi are usually present as branched, septate hyphae.

Culture

Multiple inoculations should be made on general purpose media such as malt extract or Sabouraud's dextrose agar containing antibacterial antibiotics but *not* cycloheximide, and cultures incubated at 25–30 °C (never 37 °C). Doubt as to the significance of isolates must exist in the absence of microscopical evidence, although the number of positive inocula and the association of fungal colonies with the position of the inocula may be helpful in reaching a decision.

Treatment

Topical antifungal preparations, in particular natamycin (pimaricin).

OTOMYCOSIS

In fungal infection of the outer ear (otitis external) there is scaling, pruritis and pain. Lesions are generally dry except when there is an associated bacterial infection and then there may be an offensive discharge.

The fungi usually found in this condition are those which commonly occur as saprophytes in nature; only rarely are established pathogens recovered from the external ear canal. The commonest causal agents are species of aspergilli, especially *Aspergillus niger*. It is generally accepted that the role of the fungi is that of a saprophyte, or at most a secondary invader of tissue rendered abnormal by bacterial infection or, for example, by eczema, physical injury and/or excessive accumulation of cerumen. The conditions within such abnormal ear canals form an ideal environment for fungal growth and sporing structures which may be seen with an otoscope are frequently produced in abundance.

Diagnosis is straightforward as the fungi are easy to see in material from swabs or scrapings and grow readily in culture.

Treatment can usually be satisfactorily effected with topical antifungals such as imidazole derivatives applied in a powder base or another vehicle with drying properties. Any underlying abnormality must also be treated to prevent recurrence and concurrent antibacterial therapy is indicated in mixed infections.

SUBCUTANEOUS MYCOSES

Chapter Eleven
MYCETOMA

(Synonyms: Madura foot, maduramycosis)

Mycetoma is a chronic, granulomatous infection of skin, subcutaneous tissue, fascia and bone, which most often affects the foot or hand. It may be caused by a number of actinomycetes (actinomycetoma) and true fungi (eumycetoma) and although the causal agents are widely distributed in nature throughout the world, the disease occurs most frequently in the tropical and subtropical regions of Africa, Asia and Central America.

CLINICAL FORMS

Localized swollen lesions with multiple draining sinuses are a common feature of all forms of mycetoma (Fig. 11.1) but there is some variation according to the causal organism, the duration of the disease and the site of the lesion. Although mycetoma mainly affects the limbs, infections of almost all parts of the body have been reported. The site of the lesion often reflects the hazards of particular occupations with mycetoma of the shoulders for instance occurring most frequently in burden-bearers. The disease progresses slowly and there is usually a long period of time, often years, between infection and the formation of the characteristic lesions. However, when the buttocks or trunk are infected, spread may be relatively rapid and extensive and in infections of the scalp the bones of the skull may soon become involved.

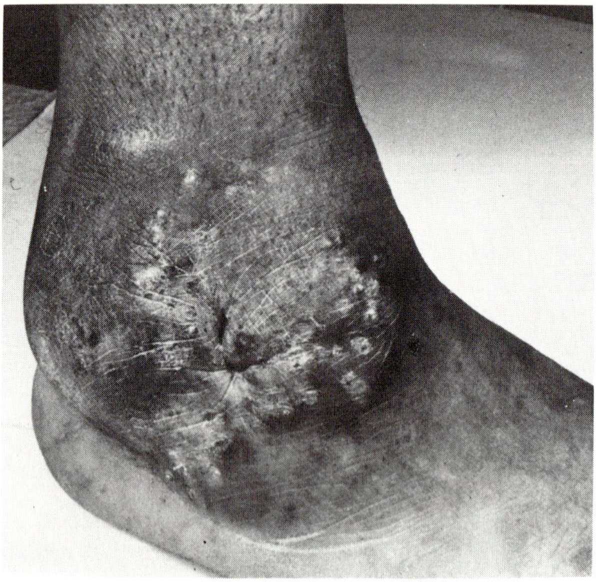

Fig. 11.1 Mycetoma of the ankle region caused by *Exophiala (Phialophora) jeanselmei*

Mycetoma is rarely a threat to life but it frequently causes severe incapacity. The prognosis differs markedly according to the causal organism; infections with actinomycetes respond well to early therapy with antibacterial agents but for eumycetoma there is no effective chemotherapy and radical surgery is usually necessary.

EPIDEMIOLOGY

Mycetoma follows subcutaneous inoculation, usually by means of a puncture wound, of one of the causal fungi or actinomycetes from a saprophytic source in soil or vegetable substrate. The distribution of the disease is strongly influenced by climate. It is most prevalent in Africa, from the Sudan westwards to Senegal, and in India, Central America and Mexico; sporadic cases occur elsewhere in the world. Within the highly endemic regions, where many of the population are scantily clad and frequently go barefoot, the importance of occupation is also clearly illustrated by the more frequent occurrence of mycetoma in males than in females and by the preponderance of infection in those in the 20–40 year age group whose occupation involves frequent minor skin injuries and close contact with soil and vegetation.

MYCOLOGY

The species of fungi and actinomycetes most frequently encountered in mycetoma are shown in Table 11.1 but this is by no means a complete list of causal agents. Clearly the range of agents is determined by their opportunistic potential together with the frequency and degree of exposure and the resistance of the host.

Table 11.1 Common causal agents of mycetoma

	Colour of grain
Eumycetoma	
Acremonium (*Cephalosporium*) *falciforme*	White
A. kiliense	White
A. recifei	White
Leptosphaeria senegalensis	Black
Madurella mycetomatis	Black
M. grisea	Black
Pseudallescheria (*Petriellidium*) *boydii*	White
Exophiala (*Phialophora*) *jeanselmei*	Black
Actinomycetoma	
Actinomadura (*Streptomyces*) *madurae*	White or yellow
A. pelletieri	Red
Nocardia brasiliensis	White
Streptomyces somaliensis	Yellow

Within the tissues of the host the causal organisms develop to form compacted colonies (grains) which vary in size from 0.5–2 mm. The shape of the grain varies considerably and the colour is determined by the characteristics of the causal agent (Table 11.1). It is relatively easy to distinguish between the grains of actinomycetoma, composed of very fine hyphae (0.5–1 μm diam.) with ill-defined cell walls, and eumycetoma grains in which the hyphae have clearly defined walls and are of much larger size (2–5 μm diam.) (Fig. 11.2). However, specific identification of the actinomycete or fungus can seldom be achieved without isolation in culture.

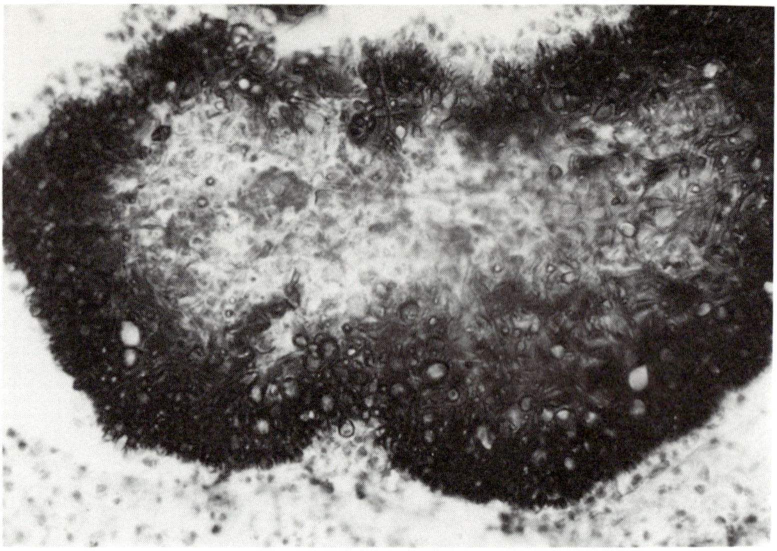

Fig. 11.2 Section of grain of *Madurella grisea* (× 270. Stained PAS)

DIAGNOSIS

Direct examination

The presence of grains in pus or other exudate is diagnostic and it is seldom necessary to stain smears since the grains are usually visible to the naked eye. However, grains should be crushed in KOH to determine their colour and to differentiate between actinomycetoma and eumycetoma. If staining is considered necessary, crushed grains should be Gram-stained; the hyphae of the actinomycetes and some of the fungi are Gram-positive. Biopsy specimens, which should be taken as deeply as possible, can also be examined in KOH but it is usually advisable to section and stain this material.

Culture

The selection of the medium and preparation of the grains for culture differs for actinomycetes and fungi and prior identification to this level by direct examination is therefore advisable. In all cases in order to minimize contamination, grains from the deepest parts of the biopsy specimen should be used; actinomycete grains should be washed in sterile saline and fungal grains in saline supplemented with antibacterial antibiotics. Grains should be crushed in the washing solution and inoculated on brain-heart infusion agar or blood agar for actinomycetes and on Sabouraud's dextrose agar (without cycloheximide) for fungi. Both media should be used if insufficient information is available from the direct microscopy. Incubation at 37°C and also at 25–30°C is recommended. Cultures should be retained for up to 6 weeks before discarding. For the identification of fungal isolates which do not sporulate, subcultures on low nutrient media may be helpful to encourage characteristic spore production.

Animal inoculation

Animal inoculation is of no diagnostic value in mycetoma.

Serology

Serological tests can be used as an aid to diagnosis of mycetoma. They are seldom necessary in overt disease because of the characteristic clinical appearance of the lesions but may be of value for the detection of early infection.

Patients with mycetoma develop precipitating antibodies to the causal organism and these can be detected by ID or CIE. Cross-reactions occur between several of the organisms involved but it is generally possible to distinguish between infections due to actinomycetes and true fungi and on occasion to identify the specific causal agent. Because of the importance of this information to prognosis and therapy, precipitin tests should be used to classify the infective agent when the results of direct microscopy and/or culture are in doubt or not available.

TREATMENT

Actinomycetoma

Antibacterial antibiotics and sulphonamides. Cotrimoxazole and rifampicin are an effective combination. Average duration of therapy is 9 months. Surgery is rarely required.

Eumycetoma

Chemotherapy is ineffective. Radical surgery is necessary.

Chapter Twelve
CHROMOMYCOSIS

(Synonym: chromoblastomycosis)

Chromomycosis is a chronic, localized disease of the skin and subcutaneous tissue most often involving the limbs and characterized by crusted and usually raised lesions. It may be caused by several dematiaceous soil fungi. The disease is mainly encountered in tropical and subtropical regions.

CLINICAL FORMS

The lesions of chromomycosis are characteristically verrucose, frequently ulcerated and may be raised up to about 3 cm with the rough irregular surfaces giving a cauliflower-like appearance (Fig. 12.1). Infection is confined to the skin and subcutaneous tissues and in most instances the condition is relatively painless. Initially lesions are solitary but slow localized spread occurs and satellite lesions also develop by autoinoculation. The lower legs and feet are most often affected but other parts of the body, especially the arms, hands, shoulders and neck, may be involved. Secondary bacterial infection may result in lymphatic obstruction and elephantiasis of the legs.

EPIDEMIOLOGY

Infection occurs by entry of the causal fungi to the cutaneous tissues through a wound. The fungi are

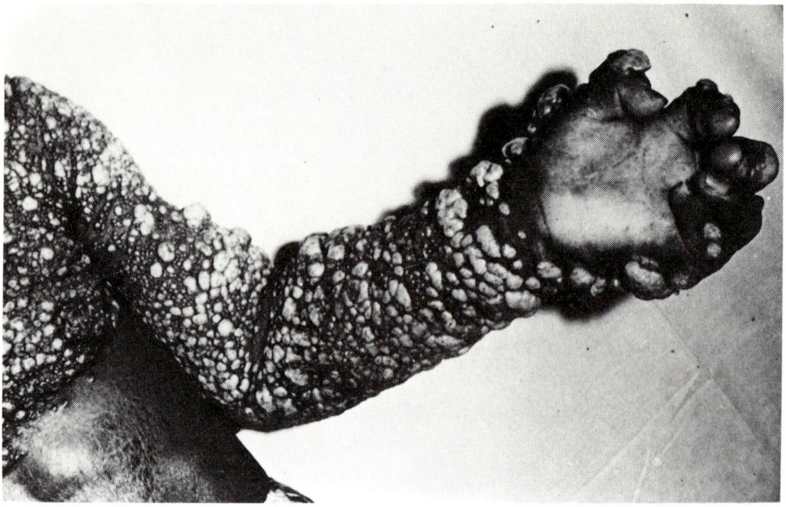

Fig. 12.1 Extensive chromomycosis of many years duration affecting arm and shoulder of native of Caribbean island

widely distributed as saprophytes in soil and decaying vegetation in all types of climates and although a single species may predominate in certain localities it is not unusual to find infections caused by other species in the same area. The disease occurs occasionally in temperate zones but it is most frequently encountered in warmer climates where individuals go barefoot and wear the minimum of clothing. Chromomycosis is very common for example in Mexico, Cuba and other parts of Latin America.

The disease occurs more often in males than in females and is more common in rural than in urban areas, reflecting the importance of the occupational risk factors.

MYCOLOGY

The causal fungi are mycelial, dematiaceous species known only in their asexual reproductive state and are morphologically very similar (Fig. 12.2). The characteristics of their asexual spore production may vary with environmental conditions and substrate and more than one method of spore formation may occur in a single isolate. There is therefore much controversy regarding their classification, and identification

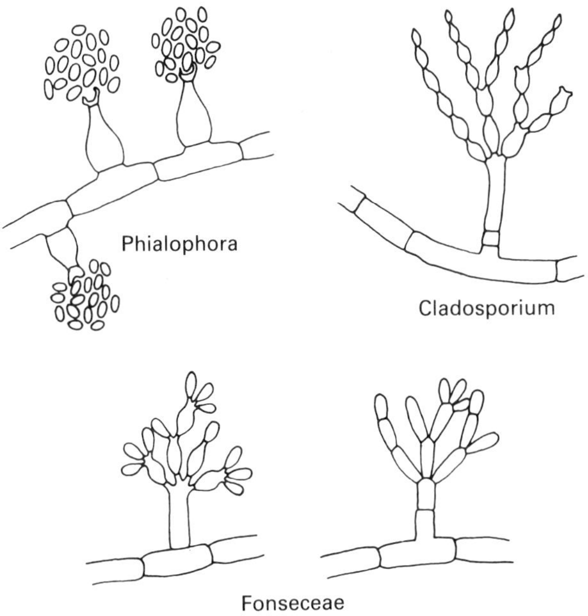

Fig. 12.2 Line drawings to illustrate the variation in form of asexual spore production by various causal agents of chromomycosis. In *Fonseceae, Phialophora* and *Cladosporium* type sporing also occurs

is difficult. Three genera, *Phialophora, Fonseceae* and *Cladosporium*, and approximately nine species are at present recognized with *F. pedrosoi, P. verrucosa, P. compacta, P. dermatitidis* and *C. carrionii* being most commonly implicated as agents of the disease.

DIAGNOSIS

Direct examination

The brown pigmented fungal structures are relatively easy to see and examination of skin scrapings and crusts from lesions in KOH usually gives satisfactory results. In such material the fungi are often present as hyphae (2–8 μm diam.) which may be distorted and swollen to a diameter of 12 μm. In pus and biopsy material from deeper tissues the fungi are present as rounded, thick-walled cells (4–12 μm diam.) occurring singly or in short chains or clusters (Fig. 12.3). These can be seen in HE preparations because of their natural brown colour but special fungi stains render them even more conspicuous.

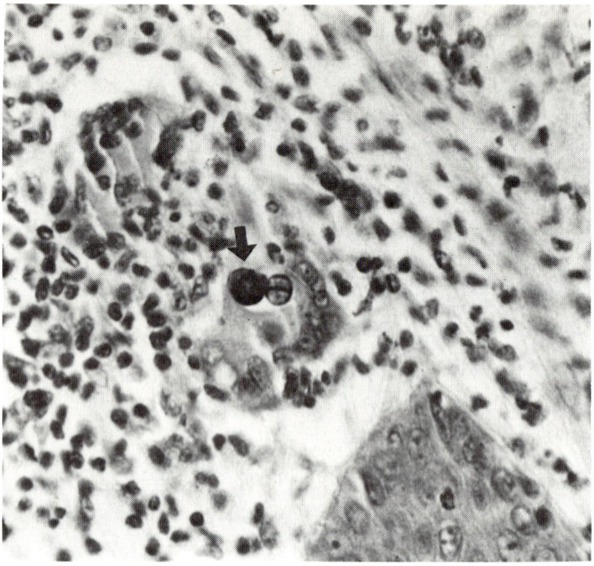

Fig. 12.3 Biopsy section showing thick-walled, dark coloured fungal cells in lesion of chromomycosis; identity of fungus unknown (× 400. Stained HE)

Culture

The fungi grow well on common isolation media such as Sabouraud's dextrose or malt extract agar and culture should always be attempted to confirm a diagnosis made on clinical grounds and/or by direct examination, especially if the latter has shown only the hyphal form of the fungus. Contamination is likely to be troublesome, especially in specimens from superficial parts of lesions and the supplementation of isolation media with antibacterial antibiotics and cycloheximide, to which the causal fungi are resistant, is advisable. Incubation should be at 25–30°C and since growth is slow, cultures should be retained for 4–6 weeks. Colonies are dark, olivaceous-grey to black, compact and usually folded or with radial grooves. The microscopical characteristics are best studied by slide culture.

Animal inoculation

Progressive infections cannot be produced in laboratory animals and animal inoculation is of no diagnostic value.

Serology

Serological tests are seldom used for the diagnosis of chromomycosis because of the ease with which the fungi are detected in readily accessible clinical material. However, somatic mycelial extracts of *F. pedrosoi* have been used to detect precipitating antibodies by ID and there are also reports of the detection of complement-fixing antibodies in patients with chromomycosis.

TREATMENT

Localized excision of solitary lesions is satisfactory in some patients. Prolonged (3–6 months) antifungal therapy is needed for most cases. Flucytosine was the drug of choice and until recently thiabendazole was second choice; oral ketoconazole is now giving promising results over a shorter (6-week) period.

PHAEOHYPHOMYCOSIS

The dematiaceous fungi that cause chromomycosis may on rare occasions, usually in compromised individuals, be responsible for opportunistic infections such as localized cystic cutaneous infection following deep inoculation of the fungus to subcutaneous tissues, or brain abscesses resulting from haematogenous spread. Although the same group of fungi is involved, these diseases are clinically distinct and cannot be considered as chromomycosis. Since the fungi are present in the tissues in hyphal form, rather than in thick-walled cell clusters, they are best described initially in general terms as phaeohyphomycosis and given a more accurate designation, for example, cerebral cladosporiosis or subcutaneous phaeomycotic cyst according to the fungus involved and the site affected. Subcutaneous forms are usually treated by localized excision but deep-seated infection requires combined therapy with intravenous amphotericin B and oral flucytosine.

Chapter Thirteen SPOROTRICHOSIS

Sporotrichosis is a subcutaneous infection which characteristically shows lymphatic spread but which may remain localized. On rare occasions the disease may disseminate widely. The causal fungus *Sporothrix schenckii* occurs as a saprophyte in soil and on vegetation. The disease has a worldwide distribution.

CLINICAL FORMS

Sporotrichosis most frequently presents as a nodular, ulcerating disease of the skin and subcutaneous tissue with spread along local lymph channels resulting in a chain of swollen lymph nodes (Fig. 13.1). Typically the primary lesion is located on the hand with secondary lesions extending along the arm. In some patients, however, perhaps related to the particular strain of *S. schenckii* or to the immunity of the individual, a lesion will remain localized or 'fixed'. Conversely, the disease occasionally may disseminate to involve the bones, joints, lungs and also, in rare instances, the central nervous system. This dissemination will usually be accompanied by the development of more widespread lesions of the skin and of the buccal and nasal mucosa. Disseminated disease, which is believed to be the result of spread from the primary cutaneous lesion rather than from a primary pulmonary focus, usually occurs in debilitated hosts such as those with pre-existing malignant disease. In most healthy individuals the immunity that develops

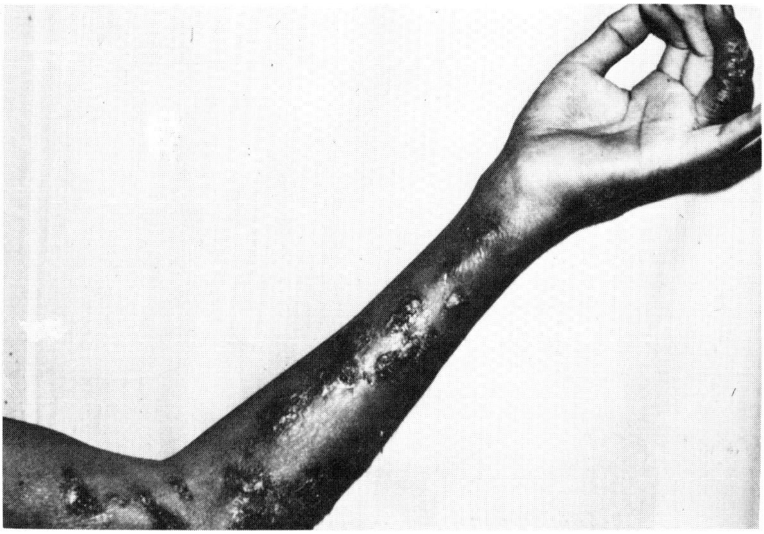

Fig. 13.1 Sporotrichosis. Typical case with chain of nodular, ulcerating lesions resulting from lymphatic spread of the disease from primary lesion on the finger

as a result of the cutaneous infection prevents further spread of the disease.

EPIDEMIOLOGY

The causal fungus has been isolated from soil and vegetation on numerous occasions and in many localities throughout the world. Infections, almost without exception, are associated with cuts, scratches or puncture wounds due to thorns and splinters in those who handle soil and plant materials and accordingly the most commonly involved sites are the hands and arms.

The disease occurs sporadically in both temperate and tropical zones but there is considerable variation in its incidence. In Mexico and certain other parts of Latin America, sporotrichosis is common, although the largest recorded epidemic, involving more then 3000 men, occurred in South African goldminers where the fungus was shown to be growing on the wooden pit-props and in surrounding soils. However, the variable occurrence of infection cannot always be directly related to the distribution of the fungus in soil or to climatic conditions.

MYCOLOGY

S. schenckii is dimorphic. In nature, and in culture at 25–30 °C, it develops as mycelium composed of thin (1–2 μm diam) septate hyphae, often lying in parallel bundles, with slender conidiophores of variable length formed at right angles and bearing clusters of thin-walled, hyaline, broadly oval spores (2–3 × 3–6 um) at the tips (Fig. 13.2). Primary isolates of *S. schenckii* may also produce dark thick-walled globose conidia often arranged in a sheath around the hyphae. The yeast phase is formed in tissue (Fig. 13.3) and at 37 °C on Sabouraud's dextrose or blood agar and is composed of spherical or cigar-shaped cells 1–3 × 3–10 μm in size.

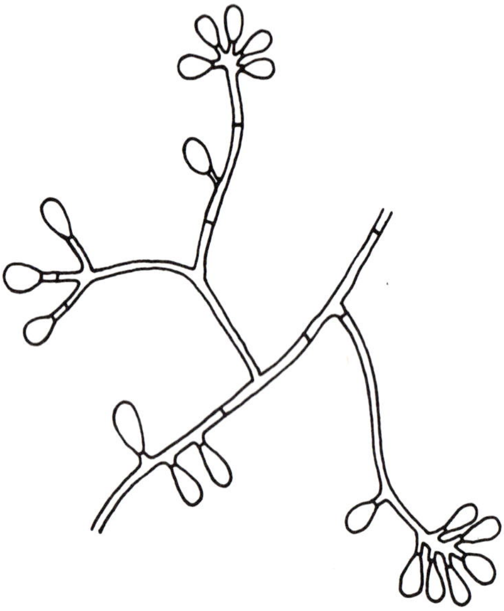

Fig. 13.2 Diagrammatic representation of asexual spore production in *Sporothrix schenckii*

Although closely associated with vegetable matter there is no evidence that *S. schenckii* is a plant pathogen. However, there is evidence to suggest that *S. schenckii* is closely related morphologically, serologically and biochemically to members of the genus *Ceratocystis* of the Ascomycotina. Species of *Ceratocystis* are widespread in nature and some such as *C. ulmi*, the cause of Dutch Elm disease, are established plant pathogens. Some *Ceratocystis* species have been

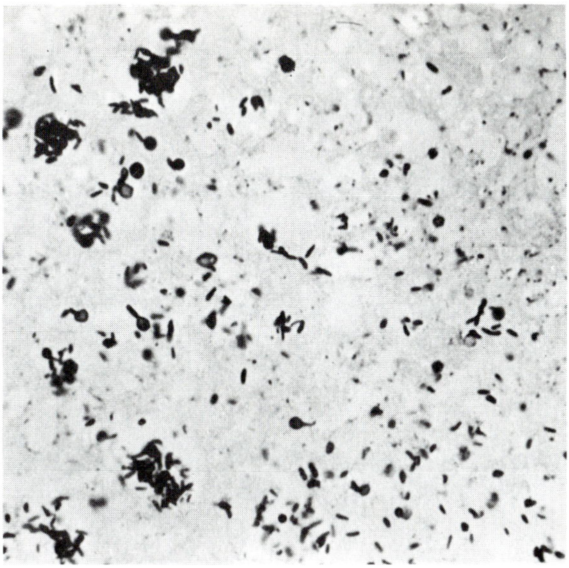

a)

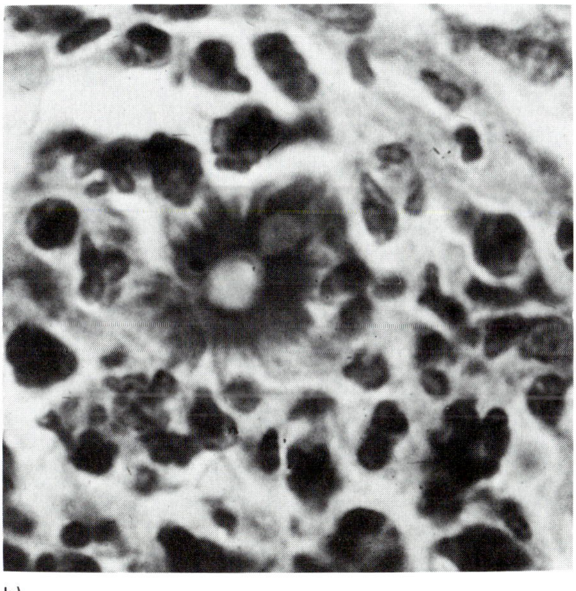

b)

Fig. 13.3 (a) The parasitic (yeast) phase of *Sporothrix schenckii* in mouse testis (× 320. Stained methenamine-silver). (b) Asteroid body. A characteristic feature of sporotrichosis in tissue. Note eosinophilic material radiating from yeast cells (× 1200. Stained HE) shown to become pathogenic for mice after serial passage and many like *S. schenckii* show dimorphism.

DIAGNOSIS

Laboratory diagnosis should be made from pus aspirated from subcutaneous nodules or from swabs of moist, ulcerated lesions. Biopsies should be avoided because the surgical procedure may spread the infection and hinder the healing of the lesion.

Direct examination

This is of little value for diagnosis because so few of the small *S. schenckii* yeast cells are present within diseased tissues and efforts should be directed mainly towards isolation in culture. Fluorescent antibody staining of clinical material with specific antiserum to the yeast cells of *S. schenckii* increases the chance of demonstrating the organism microscopically but facilities and reagents for such a procedure are seldom routinely available.

Culture

S. schenckii grows well on a wide range of culture media and the mycelial phase usually develops within 7–10 days on Sabouraud's dextrose or blood agar at 25–30 °C. Initially, the colonies appear moist and glabrous but become membranous and wrinkled with age. The colour usually changes from a cream or light brown to dark-brown or black with age but pigmentation is variable.

Confirmation of identity depends on the typical micromorphology of the mycelial phase and its conversion to the yeast phase at 37 °C.

Animal inoculation

S. schenckii causes a progressive disease in mice and rats and intraperitoneal inoculation of male animals with spores of the fungus causes orchitis within approximately 10 days. Inoculation of clinical material directly into animals is not, however, useful for diagnosis because generally too few organisms are present to initiate infection.

Immunology and serology

Skin tests

Mycelial and yeast phase antigens of *S. schenckii* have been used in skin tests but the results have been variable and specificity poor and they are not routinely used for diagnostic purposes.

Serological tests

These are very helpful in diagnosis and are especially valuable for the extracutaneous, disseminated forms of the disease which lack distinct clinical features. Although several tests are available, the WCA and LPA tests are recommended because of their sensitivity and specificity. Precipitin and CF tests give less reliable results.

The LPA test, using latex particles sensitized with yeast phase culture filtrate antigens of *S. schenckii*, has a sensitivity of over 90%. It is highly specific, gives results within a few minutes and is ideal for routine laboratory use. Titres of 1:4 or higher are considered presumptive evidence of sporotrichosis. The WCA test has a sensitivity comparable to the LPA test but it requires several hours incubation and may give false positive results, with titres ≤1:16, in patients with leishmaniasis.

The tests have little prognostic value since titres change little on successful therapy.

TREATMENT

Cutaneous form. Oral potassium iodide. Local heat may help.

Disseminated form. Intravenous amphotericin B. Oral ketoconazole has been used successfully in a few cases of early disseminated disease.

Chapter Fourteen RHINOSPORIDIOSIS

Rhinosporidiosis, caused by *Rhinosporidium seeberi*, is a chronic, granulomatous disease of the mucocutaneous tissues characterized by the production of large polyps or wart-like lesions. More than 80% of infections have been diagnosed in India and Sri Lanka.

CLINICAL FORMS

The nose is most commonly affected, followed by the conjuctiva of the eyes. Infection of other mucosal sites such as anus, vagina and ears have been reported but are rare, as are cutaneous infections except when they occur as extensions from infected mucosa. In the nose the polyps are usually pedunculated and extrude from the nostril as large pink to red cauliflower-like masses. Infections of the eye are usually unilateral and growths may be sessile or pedunculated.

EPIDEMIOLOGY

Rhinosporidiosis is not contagious but the exogenous source of infection is not exactly known. Furthermore, all attempts to isolate the fungus from lesions have failed. Circumstantial evidence indicates the existence of a natural habitat in water because of the occurrence of the disease mainly in those who regularly bathe or work in stagnant pools and also because the morphology of the parasitic phase of the fungus suggests that it belongs taxonomically to a class of fungi with motile spores adapted to an aquatic existence. It has been postulated that water insects or fish may be hosts of the fungus and the similarity of *R. seeberi* to *Ichthyosporidium*, a fungal pathogen of salmon and trout has been noted.

The disease has been diagnosed in almost all parts of the world but apart from the highly endemic areas in India and Sri Lanka the only other region where the disease occurs naturally is in South America. In most instances infections which have been diagnosed in other countries have occurred in individuals who were natives of, or had paid extended visits to an endemic region.

Most infections occur in males and in those from rural areas with close and frequent contact with fresh water pools. However, a connection between infections of the conjunctiva and the occurrence of dust storms and minor eye injuries has also been observed.

MYCOLOGY

The causal organism, *R. seeberi*, is generally accepted to be a fungus although some investigators believe it may be a sporozoan. If a fungus, it is likely to be related to genera such as *Chytridium* or *Synchytrium* which have parasitic phases in algae and higher plants closely resembling the sporangia of *R. seeberi* in man. Within the host tissue large sporangia (spherules) (<350 μm) are formed with a clearly defined wall, approximately 5 μm thick in the young developing stage but which becomes thinner and in which a pore is formed when mature (Fig. 14.1). Large numbers of spores are formed within the sporangia and these are released through the pore. The spores at the time of release measure 6–7 μm and each may develop to form a new sporangium.

DIAGNOSIS

Direct examination

Clinically and in specimens from lesions, the spor-

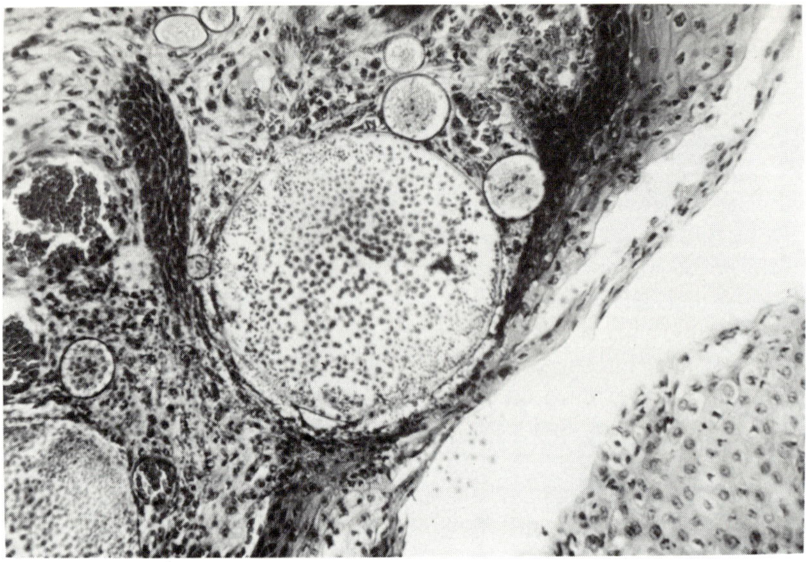

Fig. 14.1 Rhinosporidiosis. Tissue section showing a large, fully mature sporangium of *Rhinosporidium seeberi* (with numerous endospores), and several stages of sporangial development (× 140. Stained PAS)

angia may often be seen with the naked eye and both sporangia and spores can usually be easily identified microscopically in tissue macerated in KOH. Tissue sections stained with HE also show the fungal structures adequately but they are particularly prominent when stained with specific fungal stains.

Culture

Numerous attempts to culture the organism have been unsuccessful.

Animal inoculation

Although the disease occurs naturally in horses, mules and cattle, attempts at experimental infection of animals have been unsuccessful.

Immunology and serology

Little is known about the immunology of rhinosporidiosis and serological tests are not available for diagnosis.

TREATMENT

Surgical excision.

Chapter Fifteen
LOBOMYCOSIS

(Synonym: keloidal blastomycosis)

Lobomycosis is a rare, slowly progressive disease of the skin and subcutaneous tissue caused by *Loboa loboi* and in man is apparently restricted in distribution to a region stretching from Mexico southwards to Central Brazil.

CLINICAL FORMS

The infection is restricted to the dermis and neither the deeper tissues nor mucosae are involved. The lesions vary in appearance according to the duration of infection and to a lesser extent with the site involved. They occur as single, small (approx. 1 cm) nodules in the early stages and spread to become elevated and keloidal, with fresh satellite lesions appearing eventually. The most common sites of infection are the exposed areas such as the limbs and face. There is usually no discomfort to the patient although ulceration of older lesions may occur.

EPIDEMIOLOGY

All attempts to isolate the fungus from lesions of infected individuals have failed and although it is accepted that the source of infection is exogenous, the natural habitat of the causal fungus is unknown. Within the endemic area the majority of infections have been diagnosed in inhabitants of the Amazon region of Brazil and particularly among those who work in close contact with the environment in regions of dense vegetation where both humidity and temperature is high. There is no predilection for infection of any one race of people. The disease has also been diagnosed outside the endemic area in dolphins near the coast of Florida.

MYCOLOGY

The fungus is present in abundance in the dermis, usually within giant cells and macrophages, as spherical or elliptical cells which vary in size (5–12 μm diam.) (Fig. 15.1). The cell walls are clearly defined and cells are frequently seen to form small chains linked together by a thick rod-like tube. Its simple form as a pathogen gives no indication of its possible relationships with other fungi and the name *Loboa loboi*, derived from Jorge Lobo who first described the disease, is therefore generally accepted. Other generic names ascribed to the organism have arisen

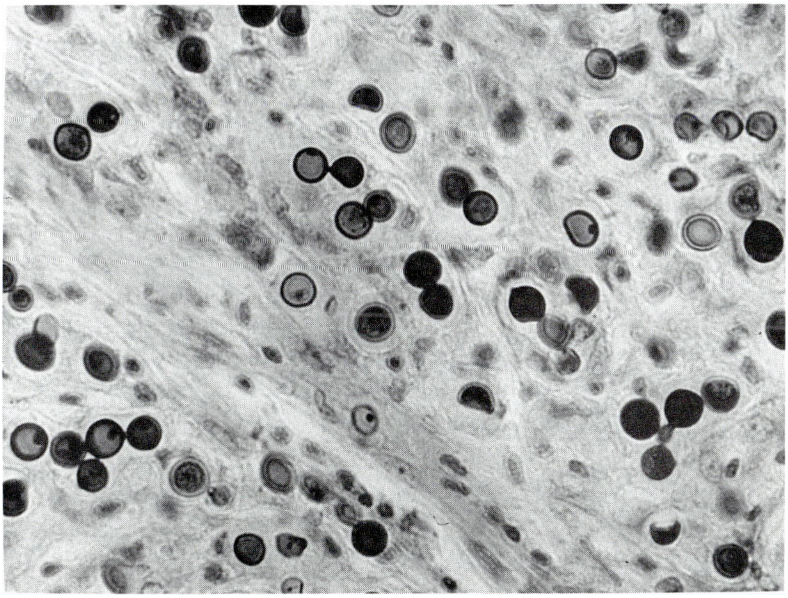

Fig. 15.1 Lobomycosis. Section of lesion showing the abundance of cells of *Loboa loboi* (× 850. Stained methenamine-silver)

from investigations in which some other fungus, usually a contaminant, has been mistaken for *L. loboi*.

DIAGNOSIS

Direct examination

Microscopical examination in KOH of material obtained by surgical excision is satisfactory for diagnosis and the numerous chains of yeast-like cells are usually easy to see. Special staining is not necessary for detection of the organism in tissue sections.

Animal inoculation

Most attempts to transfer the disease to experimental animals have been unsuccessful and, in any case, the long evolutionary period of the disease renders the procedure of little value for diagnostic purposes. It is believed that the disease may be relatively common in dolphins and it has been reported that the armadillo may probably be the animal most susceptible to experimental infection.

Immunology and serology

There are no serological procedures for the diagnosis of lobomycosis and there is no evidence that development of specific antibodies occurs in those infected or that any immunological defect predisposes to infection.

TREATMENT

Surgical excision.

SYSTEMIC MYCOSES

Chapter Sixteen COCCIDIOIDOMYCOSIS

(Synonym: valley fever)

Coccidioidomycosis, primarily an infection of the lungs caused by *Coccidioides immitis*, is a disease of major importance within endemic areas in the south-west USA and northern Mexico. In parts of the endemic regions more than 90% of inhabitants are known to have had the disease and infection rates of 20% and higher have been recorded among newcomers to these regions during their first year of residence. The majority of individuals contracting coccidioidomycosis have a self-limiting primary pulmonary illness which is often asymptomatic but a small proportion go on to develop more serious progressive and sometimes fatal secondary disease. Recovery from infection gives an immunity to reinfection which usually lasts a lifetime.

CLINICAL FORMS

Primary pulmonary disease

This form of coccidioidomycosis which develops 7–28 days after infection, is usually asymptomatic and may be marked only by conversion from a negative to a positive skin test reaction. Symptomatic pulmonary infection takes the form of an acute, influenza-like illness which is usually self-limiting. Skin rashes (erythema nodosum or erythema multiforme) develop in up to 20% of those with the primary disease, most often in adult, white females; the development of a rash indicates a good prognosis.

Benign pulmonary disease

This chronic form of the disease is characterized by the development of thin-walled, usually solitary cavities in lung tissue and is the most frequent complication of primary coccidioidomycosis. The disease may last for a number of years and become asymptomatic or it may progress to the disseminated form.

Disseminated disease

When dissemination occurs it involves virtually every tissue of the body including the central nervous system, skin and joints. It occurs in around 0.5% of those who contract the primary pulmonary disease but certain ethnic groups such as Philipinos, Negroes and American Indians are much more likely to develop this form of infection. The outlook for those with disseminated coccidioidomycosis is generally poor, particularly if there is meningeal involvement, and the overall mortality rate is around 50%.

When *C. immitis* is inoculated directly through the skin a localized subcutaneous infection results and care must be exercised to differentiate this rare, primary cutaneous infection from the more serious cases where the disease has disseminated to the skin from a pulmonary focus.

EPIDEMIOLOGY

The causal fungus *C. immitis* lives in the upper layers of the soil of semi-arid areas of southwest USA (California, Arizona, New Mexico, southwest Texas) and northern Mexico with smaller endemic areas in Central and South America. Climatic conditions, which are important in establishing the boundaries of these endemic areas, consist of a season of adequate rainfall to allow the fungus to grow, followed by a long hot, dry period during which the fungus produces large numbers of highly infectious spores which are easily dispersed in dust by recurring winds. Anyone may contract the disease but certain groups such as agricultural workers whose occupations expose them to soil dust and individuals of the dark-skinned races are especially prone to infection.

Animals may also contract the disease. On occasion symptomatic disease may develop and be diagnosed in places far removed from the American continent, usually in individuals who have visited an endemic region. Two cases were recently diagnosed in the west of Scotland in individuals who had been on holiday in California.

MYCOLOGY

C. immitis is dimorphic. The mycelial form in artificial culture and in soil produces large numbers of barrel-shaped arthrospores (4 × 6 μm diam.). These are easily dispersed in wind currents and if inhaled develop in the lungs to form spherules (30–60 μm diam.) containing numerous endospores (2–5 μm diam.). (Fig. 16.1). On rupture of the spherule wall

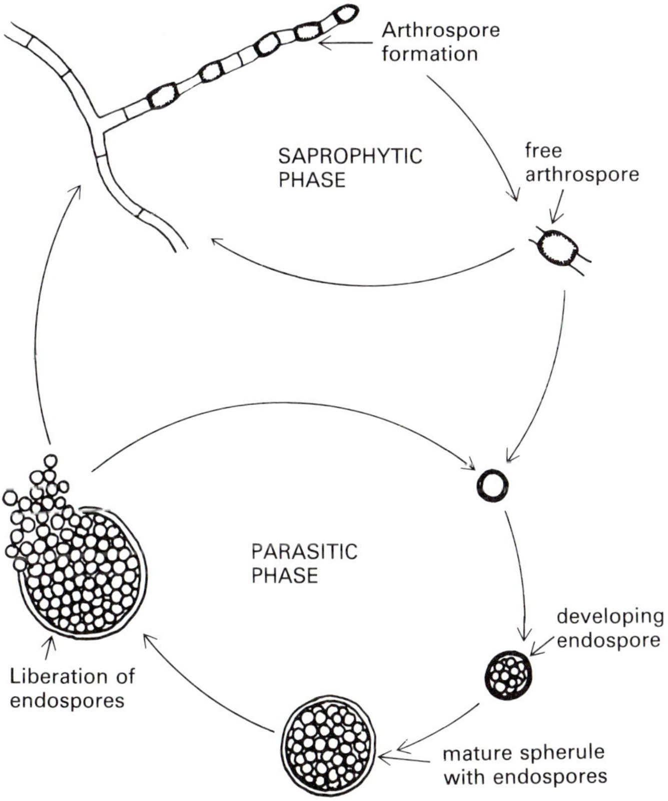

Fig. 16.1 Life cycle of *Coccidioides immitis*

the endospores develop to form new spherules in adjacent tissue or, following dissemination, in other organs of the body. When inoculated on culture media or if released into soil the endospores develop to form mycelium and arthrospores. The production of spherules in vitro requires very special growth conditions and demonstration of dimorphism is therefore unsuitable as a routine test for identification.

DIAGNOSIS

Direct examination

Microscopical examination in KOH may be very helpful in the diagnosis of coccidioidomycosis. The relatively large size and numbers of mature spherules present in sputum, pus and biopsy material makes their detection and identification in KOH mounts or in HE stained tissue sections a comparatively simple matter (Fig. 16.2). However, the smaller spherules and endospores may be difficult to differentiate from yeast cells and artifacts and for the inexperienced it is advisable to reserve most of the specimen for culture and to use special stains such as PAS for tissue sections.

Dried, heat-fixed, stained smear preparations are of no value.

Culture

Petri-dishes should never be used for the attempted isolation of the organism because of the danger of laboratory infection from the large concentrations of easily dispersed and highly infectious arthrospores. Material for culture should be inoculated on test-tube slopes of Sabouraud's dextrose agar or similar media and incubated at 25–30°C. Cultures should be maintained for at least 3 weeks before being discarded. The fungus grows relatively slowly, developing from an initially moist colony to become fluffy and within 5–12 days changes from white to pale grey or brown as arthrospores are formed. The colony form is irregular and ragged in appearance and there may be considerable variation in morphology according to strain. Mounts for microscopical examination should

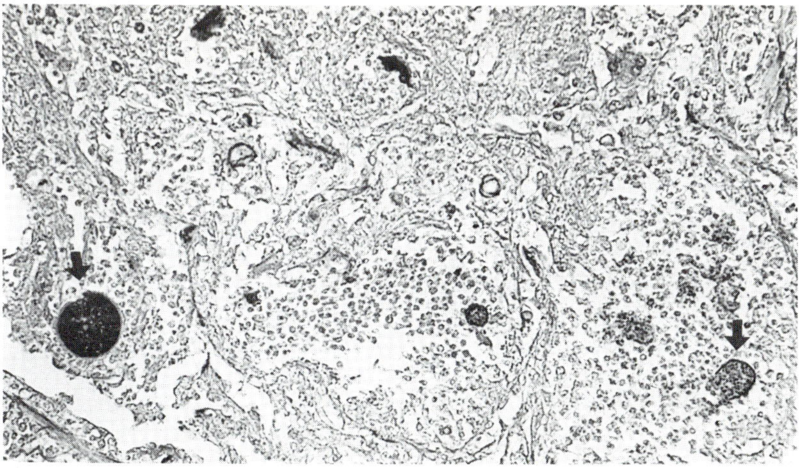

a)

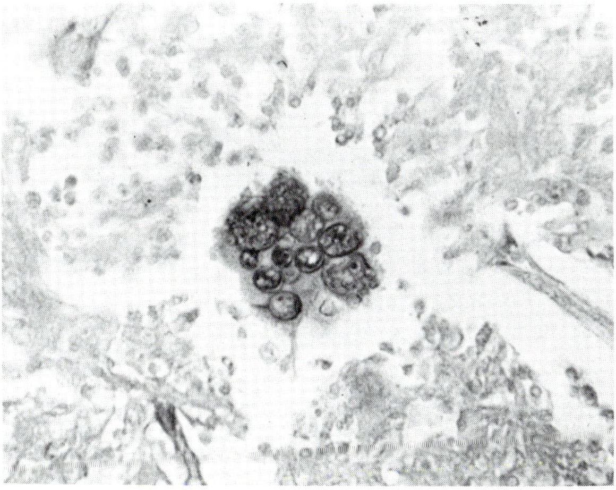

b)

Fig. 16.2 Coccidioidomycosis. Tissue sections showing parasitic phase of *Coccidioides immitis*. (a) Mature spherules with numerous endospores (× 120. Stained PAS). (b) Cluster of young spherules developing from endospores (× 450. Stained Gridley)

be made only after wetting the colony to reduce spore dispersal and will show fine, septate hyphae some of which give rise to chains of relatively thick-walled arthrospores formed from alternate cells (Fig. 16.3).

All procedures such as subculturing and the preparation of mounts for microscopy or inocula for animal infection should be carried out in a safety cabinet.

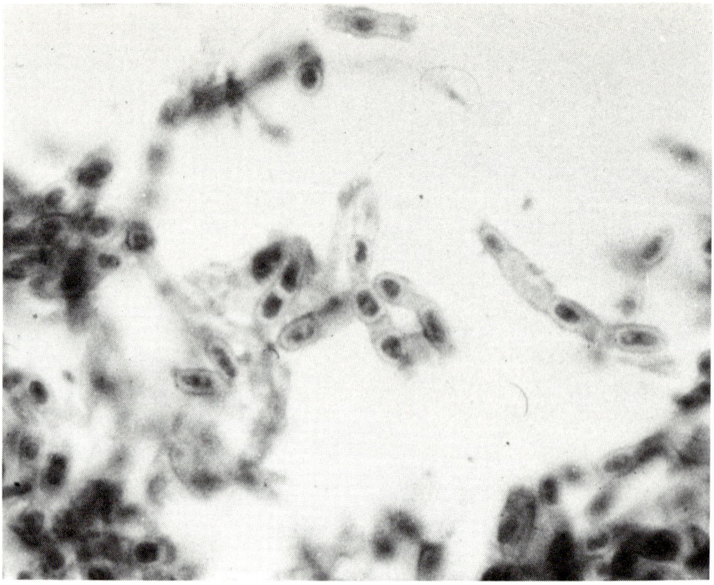

Fig. 16.3 Culture mount of *Coccidioides immitis* mycelial phase showing arthrospore formation (× 600. Cotton Blue/lactophenol)

Animal inoculation

If the identity of a culture is in doubt, and this may well be the case in laboratories in places far from the endemic regions, then animal inoculation is useful. Again this procedure should be carried out in a safety cabinet.

Mice are very susceptible to the disease and intraperitoneal inoculation of these animals with a mycelial spore suspension results in widespread infection of major organs within 1–2 weeks, with numerous lesions lining the peritoneal cavity. The presence of spherules on histopathological or KOH examination of infected material establishes the diagnosis.

Immunology and serology

Skin tests, LPA, precipitin and CF tests are used for diagnosis and for assessing prognosis in coccidioidomycosis. These are generally reliable tests although occasional cross-reactions occur in patients with histoplasmosis and blastomycosis. All tests use either coccidioidin, a culture filtrate antigen from the mycelial phase of *C. immitis*, or spherulin, an extract obtained by lysis of in vitro grown spherules of the fungus. Spherulin has become available relatively recently and results so far suggest that it is superior to coccidioidin.

Skin test

A positive skin test to extracts of *C. immitis* appears 2–21 days after the disappearance of primary symptoms. It reverts to negative in disseminated infection and a positive reaction appears only after recovery from disease. Skin testing does not elicit a humoral response as in histoplasmosis.

Precipitin test

Tests for the detection of precipitins (tube precipitation, ID or CIE) are most effective in detecting early, primary infection or exacerbation of existing disease. Precipitins usually appear 1–3 weeks after primary infection but they are short-lived, often disappearing after 4 weeks and seldom detectable after 2–6 months. In patients with disseminated coccidioidomycosis the precipitin test also becomes negative.

Latex particle agglutination

This test gives similar results to the precipitin test but is not as specific. LPA and ID are frequently used as screening tests.

Complement fixation test

Complement-fixing antibodies appear 2–3 months after infection. They are most useful for detecting disseminated disease and may never be found in patients with primary disease. In disseminated infection they persist until death or until the patient recovers. The CF titre rises as the disease progresses and declines as the patient improves. Titres as low as 1:4 or 1:8 are significant and the higher the titre the poorer the prognosis. CF tests may be carried out on serum, pleural and joint fluids.

The use of precipitin and CF tests in combination gives positive results in over 90% of patients with primary symptomatic coccidioidomycosis.

TREATMENT

Intravenous amphotericin B with concomitant intrathecal therapy in meningeal form. Miconazole and ketoconazole have been used successfully in some cases — the latter is reported to be the more promising.

Chapter Seventeen HISTOPLASMOSIS

Histoplasmosis, caused by the dimorphic fungus *Histoplasma capsulatum* is primarily a disease of the reticuloendothelial system. It most frequently occurs as an asymptomatic or relatively mild, self-limiting pulmonary infection but secondary, chronic or acute disseminated disease for which the prognosis is poor may also occur.

The majority of infections occur in the eastern parts of central USA but histoplasmosis has also been diagnosed in many different countries throughout the world.

Histoplasma is unique among pathogenic fungi in that it is an intracellular parasite.

CLINICAL FORMS

Primary pulmonary disease

Most primary infections are asymptomatic and are detected only because infected individuals develop a positive skin test reaction. However, in a significant number of cases, either because of a high degree of exposure to the fungus or because of some underlying immunological abnormality, symptoms of an acute influenza-like illness develop with fever, a non-productive cough and a chest X-ray picture resembling tuberculosis. Such infections are usually self-limiting and on recovery, patients are frequently left with discrete, calcified lesions in the lung.

In spite of the apparent limitation of the primary disease to the lungs and the mild symptoms, it is believed that the fungus becomes widely disseminated through the body by means of the reticuloendothelial system during the establishment of primary infection.

Chronic pulmonary disease

In this form of the disease, which occurs mainly in adults, large cavities develop in the lung, either directly from primary lesions or from the reactivation of previous and apparently healed pulmonary lesions. The solitary or multiple 'coin lesions' may be asymptomatic but are more often accompanied by fever, productive cough, malaise and weight loss with a clinical picture which closely resembles tuberculosis. In a proportion of cases there is further progression to give serious, acute generalized disease.

Disseminated disease

A small proportion of individuals develop a serious, acute progressive form of the disease. There is widespread infection of the reticuloendothelial system and any organ of the body may become involved. It is characterized by malaise, fever, weight loss and enlargement of the liver and spleen and frequently there is ulceration of the mouth and intestines. The rate of progression of the disease varies considerably from patient to patient but generally the prognosis is poor.

This type of infection occurs most often in old age or infancy and in individuals with impaired immune responses caused by underlying disease such as malignancy or by immunosuppressive therapy. It may also develop when a particularly heavy exposure to the fungus causes an infection that overwhelms the natural host defence mechanism.

A chronic, disseminated form of histoplasmosis is also recognized in which the emergence of clinical disease occurs many years after the individual contracts the infection.

EPIDEMIOLOGY

The natural habitat of *H. capsulatum* is soil enriched

with the droppings of birds or bats. Infections result from the inhalation of spores and although the disease usually occurs sporadically, focal outbreaks of infection have been documented following group exposure associated with soil disturbance of old chicken runs or starling roosts and exploration of bat-infested caves. Bats are naturally infected with *Histoplasma* as are many domestic animals, especially cats and dogs, but there is no evidence that birds become infected or serve as carriers.

The major endemic areas for histoplasmosis are the Mississippi and Ohio river valleys of the eastern USA. The incidence of infection among the population, estimated by skin testing, may be as high as 95% and it has been suggested that the high concentration of starlings in these regions and their habitual congregation in great numbers to roost is an important aetiological factor. Histoplasmosis has also been reported from a number of other parts of the USA and is known to occur in many other temperate and tropical areas throughout the world, including Central and South America, Africa, Australia, the Far-East and Europe.

MYCOLOGY

H. capsulatum is dimorphic, growing in soil and in artificial culture at 25–30 °C as septate mycelium and as an intracellular yeast in animal tissues. The yeast phase cells (2–3 × 3–4 μm) can also be produced in vitro by culture at 37 °C on blood agar or other enriched media containing cystine or cysteine. The mycelial phase usually produces two types of unicellular asexual spores. Large round, tuberculate (8–14 μm diam.) macroaleuriospores are most prominent (Fig. 17.1) but smaller broadly elliptical smooth-walled microaleuriospores (2–4 μm diam.) are also present in primary isolates.

The sexual, or perfect state of *H. capsulatum*, *Emmonsiella capsulata* is known but since it is heterothallic and formed only when the compatible '+' and '−' mating strains are brought together under particular nutritional and environmental conditions, it is unlikely to be encountered in a routine diagnostic laboratory. Although both mating strains are equally

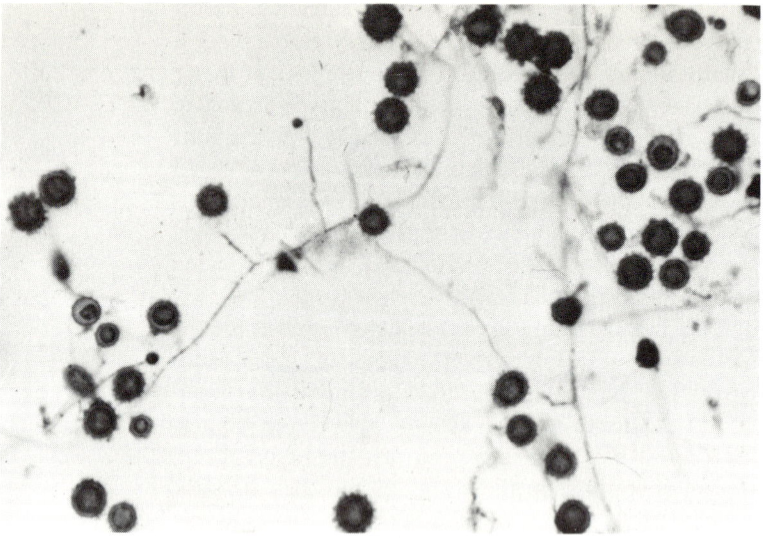

Fig. 17.1 Culture mount of *Histoplasma capsulatum* showing macroaleuriospore production (× 300. Cotton Blue/lactophenol)

prevalent in soil there is some evidence that the disease is caused more frequently by the '−' mating strain.

The cleistothecium of *E. capsulata* is buff-coloured and globose (80–250 μm diam.) with a peridium of net-like hyphae which encloses a radiate mass of tightly coiled hyphae and numerous groups of asci. The ascospores (1.5 μm diam.), 8 per ascus, are pyriform and hyaline with smooth walls.

DIAGNOSIS

Direct examination

Examination of specimens such as sputum or pus in KOH, which is satisfactory for many other fungal diseases, is unsatisfactory and all material should be examined as stained smears. Smears should be fixed with methyl alcohol and stained with either the Wright or Giemsa procedure; overstaining may be helpful since it emphasizes the fungus. For tissue sections staining by PAS, Gridley or methenamine-silver is satisfactory. The diagnostic feature is the presence of the small oval yeast cells (2–3 × 3–4 μm) packed within macrophages or monocytes (Fig. 17.2), although a number of yeasts liberated by rupture of

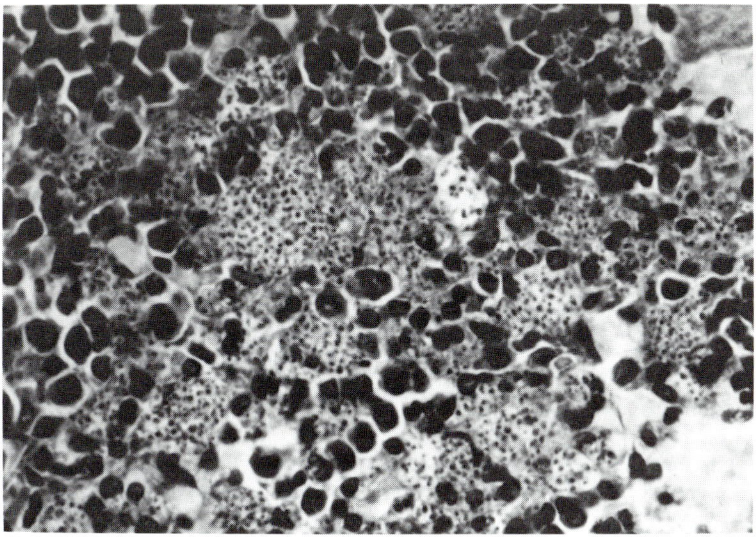

Fig. 17.2 Histoplasmosis. Tissue showing parasitic phase of *Histoplasma capsulatum*: numerous small oval yeast cells within macrophages (× 400. Stained PAS)

the host cells are also present. A characteristic of *H. capsulatum* is that the fixation procedure frequently results in shrinkage of the fungal cytoplasm away from the yeast cell wall giving a clear area which resembles a narrow capsule.

Culture

Specimens should be cultured on Sabouraud's dextrose agar at 25–30 °C to obtain the mycelial phase of *H. capsulatum*. These cultures represent a laboratory hazard and for reasons of safety, test-tube slopes rather than petri-dishes should be used for isolation. Mycelial colonies may develop rather slowly (1–4 weeks) and cultures should be retained for up to 6 weeks before discarding. Initially the colonies are fluffy and either white or buff-brown and both types may be isolated from the same patient. The brown colonies commonly show sectoring and conversion to the white type.

Culture at 37 °C on enriched media such as glucose-cysteine-blood agar results in the development of the yeast phase but this is not recommended for primary isolation since the mycelial phase is much easier to recover and identify. However, mycelial to yeast conversion by culture at 37 °C on enriched media is useful to confirm the identity of isolates.

Animal inoculation

Mice are very susceptible to histoplasmosis and intraperitoneal inoculation can be used both for primary isolation or to confirm the identity of an isolate. For isolation from clinical material or soil/faeces the inoculation should be supplemented with adequate antibacterial antibiotics and for identification of isolates a large dose (10^7 viable units or more) is recommended. In both cases specimens of spleen and liver should be examined histologically and by culture after 2 weeks or on earlier death of the animals.

Immunology and serology

Skin tests

Skin tests with histoplasmin, a culture filtrate antigen from the mycelial phase of *H. capsulatum*, have been used widely to identify the endemic areas of histoplasmosis. A positive skin test indicates past or present infection. It does not, however, distinguish between them and a negative test does not exclude infection. Skin tests are not recommended for diagnostic purposes because they induce a humoral antibody response which makes the interpretation of subsequent serodiagnostic tests difficult. Blood for serology should therefore be taken either before or within 2–3 days of skin testing.

Serological tests

These are often the basis for a definitive diagnosis of histoplasmosis, although cross-reactions can occur, mainly with blastomycosis and coccidioidomycosis. Three tests (CF, ID and LPA) are commonly used, often in combination.

Complement fixation test. CF tests with histoplasmin or killed whole-yeast cells as antigen are the most widely used and give positive results in up to 96% of culturally proven cases. Yeast-phase antigens are the most sensitive and useful for screening active cases giving positive results within 2–4 weeks after first exposure to the organism. The development of antibodies to mycelial phase antigen (histoplasmin) occurs later.

Generally titres of 1:8 or more are regarded as presumptive evidence of infection, and titres of 1:32 or above indicate active disease. Titres lower than 1:8 do not, however, exclude infection — negative results are sometimes obtained in patients with primary pulmonary or advanced disseminated diseaase.

Rising CF titres (fourfold) indicate progressive disease whereas a drop in titre indicates recovery from infection although complement-fixing antibodies may persist for some time after the patient is cured.

Precipitin test. ID is a useful screening test for histoplasmosis. Precipitins appear earlier in the course of infection than complement fixing antibodies and there are also fewer problems with cross-reactions. The test, using histoplasmin antigen, gives positive results in up to 85% of infected patients. There are two major precipitin bands of diagnostic significance, namely the H and M bands. The H band indicates active infection and the M band either indicates infection (acute or chronic) or a previous skin test with histoplasmin. The M band appears first and provides early presumptive evidence of infection in patients who have not previously been skin tested.

The ID test gives only qualitative data and positive results should be confirmed by a CF test.

Latex particle agglutination The LPA test, using histoplasmin antigen, is useful for detecting acute histoplasmosis and like the ID test can be used with anticomplementary sera. Titres of 1:16 or more are considered presumptive evidence of infection. However, patients with chronic histoplasmosis can give negative results and in general the LPA test is of less value than CF and ID tests.

TREATMENT

Intravenous amphotericin B. Ketoconazole has been used successfully in a few cases.

AFRICAN HISTOPLASMOSIS

(*Histoplasma duboisii*)

This disease differs from classical histoplasmosis in distribution, being mainly restricted to the continent of Africa. It differs also clinically in that it is primarily a disease of the cutaneous and subcutaneous tissues with little evidence of pulmonary involvement. The causal fungus is morphologically identical to *H. capsulatum* in its mycelial phase but differs in that the yeast phase, in vivo and in vitro, has larger cells (12 — 15 μm diam.). Some authorities considered that *H. duboisii* is a variety of *H. capsulatum*. Treatment is as for histoplasmosis.

Chapter Eighteen BLASTOMYCOSIS

(Synonym: North American blastomycosis)

Blastomycosis, caused by *Blastomyces dermatitidis*, is a chronic infection originating in the lungs which may spread to involve other tissues, notably skin and bone. The disease occurs mainly in the North American continent. If left untreated the disease is slowly progressive and has a poor prognosis.

CLINICAL FORMS

There are three main forms of the disease which in general are characterized by suppurative and granulomatous lesions.

Primary pulmonary disease

Although symptoms are relatively mild, primary pulmonary blastomycosis is usually symptomatic and within a few weeks of infection the disease becomes chronic and may disseminate to other tissues. The chest X-ray picture can resemble that of tuberculosis or carcinoma.

Disseminated disease

In disseminated infection the chronic pulmonary disease persists and spread occurs to most organs and body tissues including bone, with formation of abscesses and granulomatous lesions.

Cutaneous disease

Chronic cutaneous disease occurs in about 80% of patients with pulmonary infection and these secondary skin lesions are a characteristic feature of blastomycosis. The skin lesions are typically raised and crusty with a well demarcated edge. It is from these characteristic lesions that the diagnosis is most often made.

Primary cutaneous infection as a result of direct inoculation of *B. dermatitidis* to the cutaneous tissues is rare and produces a localized, self-limiting lesion.

EPIDEMIOLOGY

It is accepted that infection results from inhalation of spores but the natural habitat of the causal fungus has not been established with certainty. It has been isolated from soil on only a very few occasions and experimental work indicates that the fungus is capable of survival in soil for only very short periods of time. Most infections appear to be contracted during cool wet climatic conditions and these may be related to the conditions necessary for growth and/or sporulation of the fungus in the environment.

The endemic areas for blastomycosis, based on the occurrence of human and animal infections, are the eastern, central and mid-western states of the USA and eastern Canada. A number of infections have also been diagnosed in South America and Africa. Cases of blastomycosis are sporadic and there is no convincing evidence of occupational predisposition. The highest incidence of infection is found in individuals between the ages of 30 and 50, with males more often infected than females.

In contrast to other systemic mycoses such as histoplasmosis and coccidioidomycosis, there is no clear evidence for the frequent occurrence of a mild, self-limiting, subclinical form of the disease. However, since there is no satisfactory skin test for investigative epidemiological work this possibility cannot be excluded.

MYCOLOGY

B. dermatitidis is a dimorphic fungus. Cultures of the

mycelial phase at 25–30 °C vary in texture from floccose to glabrous and from white to brown in colour. The number of spores produced is also very variable. The asexual, unicellular aleuriospores are borne on lateral branches of variable length (Fig. 18.1); they range in size from 2–10 μm in diameter and a proportion may be dumb-bell-shaped (double spores). In tissue, or in culture at 37 °C, the fungus grows as yeast cells (8–15 μm diam.) which characteristically form broad-based buds from a single pole on the mother cell. The sexual reproductive state, *Ajellomyces dermatitidis* of the Ascomycotina, is known but its production requires special cultural conditions and the presence of both '+' and '−' mating strains. The

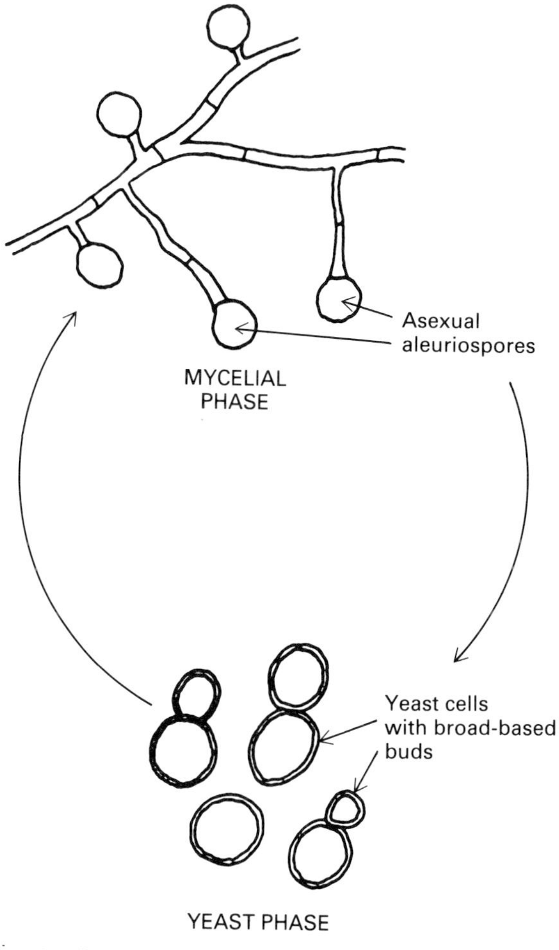

Fig. 18.1 Growth phases of *Blastomyces dermatitidis*

cleistothecium produced is morphologically very similar to that of *Emmonsiella capsulata* (the sexual state of *H. capsulatum*) and some workers believe that *Ajellomyces* and *Emmonsiella* are generic synonyms.

Blastomycosis is apparently not caused predominantly by one mating strain of *A. dermatitidis*, as is the case for histoplasmosis and *E. capsulata*.

DIAGNOSIS

Direct examination

Pus or scrapings from skin lesions, sputum from patients with suspected pulmonary infections or other appropriate clinical material can be satisfactorily examined by emulsifying in KOH. The yeast cells are thick-walled and 8–15 μm in diameter with occasional cells as large as 30 μm. The characteristic feature is the broad base (4–5 μm) bud attachment, with buds remaining attached until they are almost the same size as the mother cell, often forming chains of 3–4 cells. In biopsy material the yeast cells can usually be seen by careful examination of HE stained sections but PAS or methenamine-silver stains show them more clearly.

Culture

Sabouraud's dextrose or blood agar supplemented with antibacterial antibiotics are suitable media for the isolation of *B. dermatitidis*. The fungus is sensitive to cycloheximide and this agent should not be used in isolation media. Incubation at 25–30 °C results in the development of the mycelial phase but cultures develop rather slowly and should be retained for at least 6 weeks before discarding. Because of this prolonged incubation period and also for reasons of safety, it is advisable to use test-tube slopes rather than petri-dishes for culture. The mycelial phase cultures vary considerably in morphology and since neither the macro-nor micromorphological features are characteristic for the species, identification is usually confirmed by subculturing at 37 °C to convert to the yeast phase.

Animal inoculation

Intraperitoneal inoculation of mice with either the mycelial or yeast phase produces micro-abscesses in the peritoneal cavity after 3–4 weeks and this may be used to confirm pathogenicity of doubtful isolates.

Immunology and serology

Skin tests and serological investigations are of only limited diagnostic value because of cross-reactions with histoplasmosis and coccidioidomycosis and also because there is a relatively high proportion of non-reactors. Blastomycin, a culture filtrate antigen from the mycelial phase is used in skin tests and yeast phase antigen for CF and precipitin tests. In the CF test a titre of 1:8 or higher is considered positive but specificity is poor and, moreover, approximately 50% of those with proven blastomycosis give negative results. However, if positive, a series of CF tests showing a high or rapidly rising titre is most significant. The precipitin test, when performed with reference sera as controls, gives more specific results and up to 80% of those infected with *B. dermatitidis* give a positive result. Precipitating antibodies disappear slowly after successful therapy and can be used as a prognostic indicator.

TREATMENT

Intravenous amphotericin B. Hydroxystilbamidine is used in localized disease or if amphotericin B fails or proves too toxic. Ketoconazole is being evaluated.

Chapter Nineteen
PARACOCCIDIOIDO-MYCOSIS

(Synonym: South American blastomycosis)

Paracoccidioidomycosis is a chronic, granulomatous disease which may involve the lungs, mucosa, skin and lymphatic system. It is caused by the dimorphic fungus *Paracoccidioides brasiliensis* and is endemic to South and Central America. Untreated infections are progressive and have a fatal outcome.

CLINICAL FORMS

The disease most often presents as an ulcerative, granulomatous infection of the oral and nasal mucosa and the adjacent skin. These conspicuous superficial lesions are considered to be secondary to a chronic primary pulmonary infection. Other body sites such as the lymphatic system, spleen, intestines, adrenals and liver are also frequently involved. Primary cutaneous or mucosal lesions may occur but are rare. There is evidence that there may be latent infection for long periods before overt disease develops.

It is believed that, as for histoplasmosis and coccidioidomycosis, a mild self-limiting pulmonary form of paracoccidioidomycosis exists but skin tests are unreliable and this has not been confirmed.

EPIDEMIOLOGY

It is now accepted that *P. brasiliensis* usually enters the body by the respiratory tract. Circumstantial evidence clearly indicates that the fungus exists as a saprophyte in nature although isolations from extra-human sources have been made on only two occasions — from the intestinal contents of a Greater Fruit bat in Columbia and from a soil sample in Argentina. Within the endemic areas of South and Central America the disease is most frequently encountered in regions classified as subtropical mountain forests but the exact ecological niche of the fungus has yet to be found.

The highest incidence of clinical disease occurs in males, especially rural workers between 20 and 50 years of age.

MYCOLOGY

P. brasiliensis is dimorphic, growing in the mycelial phase in culture at 25–30 °C, and in the yeast phase as a pathogen or at 37 °C on complex media such as brain-heart infusion or blood agar (Fig. 19.1). Mycelial colonies are slow-growing and of variable morphology but the majority are white, velvety to floccose in texture and with a pale brown reverse. Sporulation varies with the strain and the culture medium but is usually sparse and best seen in old (8–10 week) cultures. Aleuriospores, chlamydospores and arthrospores may be formed but none are characteristic for the species and identification depends on conversion of mycelial cultures to the yeast phase. The yeast cells are oval or globose, very variable in size (2–30 μm diam.) and in pure culture regularly exhibit characteristic multipolar budding with small buds, attached by a narrow neck, encircling the mother cell (Fig. 19.2).

DIAGNOSIS

Direct examination

Microscopical examination in KOH of sputum or pus and crusts from granulomatous lesions will usually reveal yeast cells of greatly varying size (2–30 μm diam.). However, these are usually present as single cells or chains of cells and often cannot be differen-

Fig. 19.1 Growth phases of *Paracoccidioides brasiliensis*

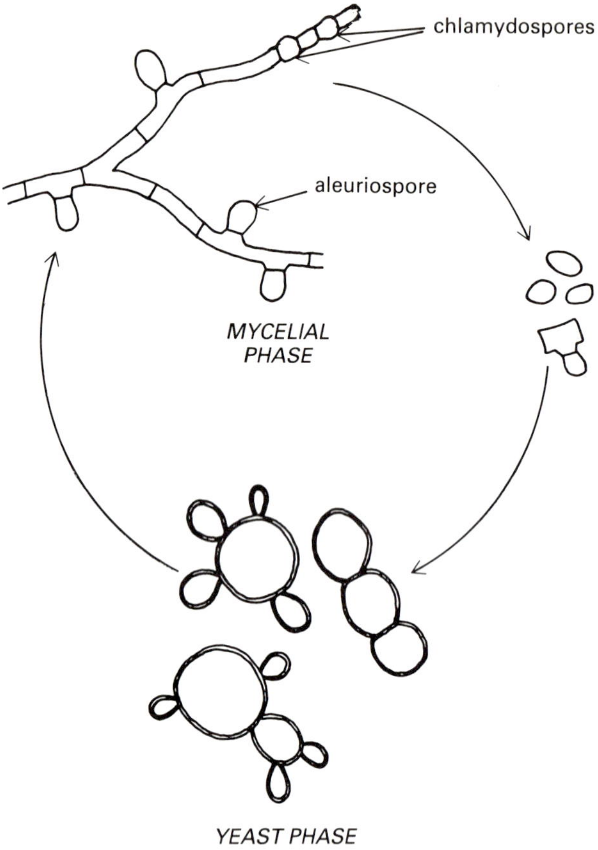

Fig. 19.2 Culture mount of yeast phase of *Paracoccidioides brasiliensis* showing characteristic multipolar budding (× 530. Cotton Blue/lactophenol)

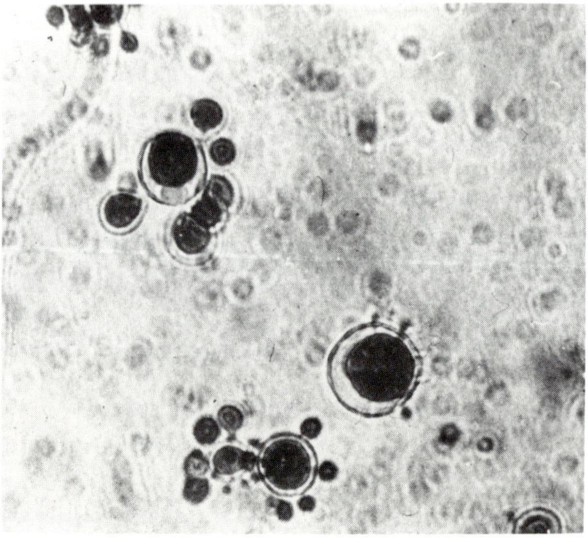

tiated from those of other fungal pathogens since the characteristic multipolar budding occurs infrequently in clinical material.

Tissue sections should be stained by methenamine-silver or PAS procedures and especially in the absence of culture a careful search made for the characteristic peripheral budding forms.

Culture

The development of both the mycelial and the yeast phase of *P. brasiliensis* is slow and cultures should be retained for at least 6 weeks before being discarded. Blood agar incubated at 37 °C is recommended for isolation of the yeast phase and agar media supplemented with yeast extract at 25–30 °C for the mycelial phase. The yeast phase is sensitive to cycloheximide and this antibiotic should not be used to supplement isolation media. It is best to confirm the identity of mycelial isolates by mycelial to yeast phase conversion. In any case this can usually be accomplished some time before adequate sporulation of the mycelial phase is likely to occur.

Animal inoculation

Natural infection of animals with *P. brasiliensis* is not known. The fungus is not highly virulent for laboratory animals and although systemic infections have been produced experimentally in mice, rabbits, guinea pigs and hamsters, these were only achieved with considerable difficulty.

Animal inoculation is not usually necessary for diagnosis but if required, pathogenicity of isolates can be confirmed by the production of orchitis in guinea pigs following intratesticular inoculation.

Immunology and serology

Skin tests

These are of limited diagnostic value because of negative reactions in a significant proportion of individuals with advanced disease and also because of cross-reactions in patients with histoplasmosis and sporotrichosis.

Serological tests

ID and CF tests are useful for diagnosis of infection and for monitoring the response to therapy. Precipitins appear first followed by complement-fixing antibodies. The ID and CF tests, using culture filtrate antigens from the yeast phase, give positive results in up to 95% and 80% respectively of patients with paracoccidioidomycosis but when used in combination diagnostic sensitivity rises to around 98%. CF titres of 1:8 or more indicate infection; high titres occur in patients with pulmonary lesions or disseminating disease whereas lower titres are associated with localized disease or occur in patients with involvement of the reticuloendothelial system. Cross-reactions are rare, particularly for the ID test, but can occur at low titres in patients with histoplasmosis. A more accurate interpretation of the ID test is possible if regard is paid to the particular precipitin lines that develop.

Antibodies decline on successful therapy. Precipitins disappear first followed by complement-fixing antibodies, although antibodies at low titres may persist for a long time after cure of the infection.

TREATMENT

Ketoconazole is emerging as the drug of choice. Intravenous amphotericin B and/or sulphonamides are also used.

Chapter Twenty CRYPTOCOCCOSIS

Cryptococcosis, caused by the capsulated yeast *Cryptococcus neoformans*, is most frequently recognised as an infection of the central nervous system (c.n.s.). It is, however, primarily a disease of the lungs which in a proportion of cases disseminates, usually to the brain. Cryptococcosis occurs sporadically throughout the world and *Cr. neoformans* has been isolated from bird droppings and soil in many countries.

CLINICAL FORMS

Pulmonary disease

Pulmonary infection with *Cr. neoformans* has no clear diagnostic features. Lesions frequently take the form of small discrete nodules ($\leqslant$1.5 cm) which often develop subpleurally. These may heal without a residual scar or they may become enlarged, encapsulated and chronic (cryptococcoma) and appear on chest X-ray as coin lesions several cm in diameter. An acute pneumonic type of disease has also been reported which radiologically appears as diffuse areas of infiltration.

It is believed that a mild, self-limiting pulmonary infection which usually goes undiagnosed is common but the absence of a specific skin test for cryptococcosis precludes confirmation.

Disseminated disease

The high frequency of infections which involve only the c.n.s. indicates that *Cr. neoformans* has a predilection for this tissue. The most familiar form of the disease is a chronic meningitis or meningoencephalitis which develops insidiously with symptoms which include headaches of increasing frequency and severity and a low grade pyrexia, followed by changes in mental state, anorexia, visual disturbances and eventually coma. The course of the disease is usually relatively rapid, although its duration can vary from a few months to many years. The outcome is always fatal if the disease is left untreated.

Although predominantly a disease of the c.n.s., lesions of the skin, mucosa, viscera and bones may also occur in disseminated cryptococcosis. Skin lesions appear as papules, pustules or as subcutaneous abscesses which may ulcerate and involvement of the bones and joints is usually associated with a painful swelling of the affected areas. In its disseminated form, cryptococcosis may resemble tuberculosis.

On rare occasions, lesions of the skin and bones with no apparent involvement of other sites have been reported and these are presumed to be the result of direct implantation of *Cr. neoformans* to these sites.

EPIDEMIOLOGY

Cr. neoformans has been recovered from the excreta of both wild and domesticated birds and from soil enriched with bird droppings in almost every country of the world. The relationship between the fungus and pigeons has been the most extensively studied because of the prevalence of these birds in urban areas and their close association with man. Isolations of *Cr. neoformans* have been made from pigeon droppings in exposed locations but the fungus is found most often in old accumulations of faeces in sheltered sites such as church towers and derelict buildings. Counts of up to 50 million viable *Cryptococcus* cells per gram dry weight of faeces have been recorded.

The association of *Cr. neoformans* with bird droppings has largely been explained by the fact that they contain nitrogenous compounds, notably creatinine, which favour the growth of the yeast. The birds themselves do not appear to become infected, possibly because of their high body temperature, although they may carry the organism in their crops.

Cr. neoformans can be divided into four serotypes (A, B, C, D). Serotypes A and D cause the vast majority of infections and it is these serotypes that have been found to be prevalent in bird droppings. Clearly, therefore, exposure to bird droppings containing the yeast poses the most significant risk to man. However in certain regions, for example in parts of California, B and C serotypes account for around 50% of cryptococcal infections and the source of these organisms has yet to be discovered.

Although infections usually occur sporadically, there are reports that outbreaks of pulmonary cryptococcosis (pneumonitis) may have occurred following group exposure to bird droppings, for example among workmen clearing accumulations of pigeon excreta.

The disease has been diagnosed more often in males than females and it is predominantly a disease of adults; there is no apparent racial predilection. The disseminated disease is known to occur most frequently in compromised patients such as those with Hodgkin's disease, sarcoidosis, collagen disease, neoplasms, or Acquired Immune Deficiency Syndrome (AIDS) and in patients treated with systemic corticosteroid drugs.

MYCOLOGY

The cells of *Cr. neoformans* are round (4–10 μm diam.) and reproduce by the production of daughter cells (buds) at any point on the cell surface. The cells are surrounded by a mucopolysaccharide capsule, the width of which varies with the strain from very narrow (<0.5 μm) up to several times the diameter of the cell. Generally the largest capsules are produced in tissue, and in vitro, the width of the capsule varies depending on the growth medium. Capsule production is greatest on rich media such as brain heart infusion or on media supplemented with thiamine when the fungus appears as creamy-white to yellow-brown mucoid colonies. However, isolates that are inherently poorly encapsulated develop as dry colonies. Under normal circumstances *Cr. neoformans* does not produce mycelium or pseudomycelium.

Within recent years it has been shown that the yeast *Cr. neoformans* is the imperfect stage of two varieties of *Filobasidiella neoformans* of the Basidiomycotina. *F. neoformans* var. *neoformans* and *F. neoformans* var. *gattii* are heterothallic and their mating strains conform to the four serotypes (A, B, C, D) of *Cr. neoformans*. Serotypes A and D are the compatible mating strains of *F. neoformans* var. *neoformans* and serotypes B and C those of *F. neoformans* var. *gattii*. Conjugation of two compatible yeast cells results in the development of septate hyphal growth with the formation of clamp connections, a characteristic feature of the Basidiomycotina. Slender, club-shaped basidia are borne terminally on the aerial hyphae and give rise to basidiospores which develop to produce new yeast cells. The two varieties differ mainly in the form of the basidiospores, those of var. *neoformans* are oval to subglobose with finely roughened walls whereas those of var. *gattii* are rod-shaped and smooth.

DIAGNOSIS

Pulmonary cryptococcosis usually goes undiagnosed and the clinical diagnosis of c.n.s. infections also presents difficulties since it produces clinical and pathological changes that may resemble other infections such as tubercular or syphilitic meningitis, brain tumours and certain forms of severe mental disorder. Diagnosis depends on the demonstration of *Cr. neoformans* in cerebrospinal fluid (c.s.f.) or other material either by direct microscopy or culture or by serological tests for the detection of cryptococcal antigen.

Direct examination

Cryptococcus can be seen in unstained preparations of c.s.f. by mixing a drop of spinal fluid or a portion of centrifuged deposit in a drop of nigrosine or India ink. Microscopical examination under a low light

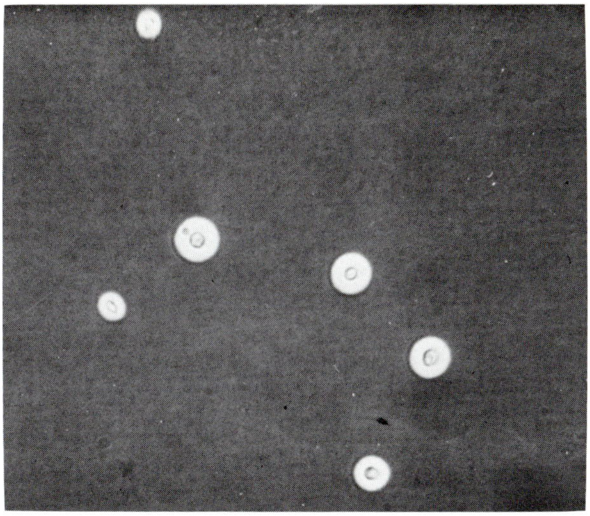

Fig. 20.1 Slide mount of *Cryptococcus neoformans* in India ink showing well-defined capsules (× 100)

intensity shows the distinctive capsule of *Cr. neoformans* as a clear halo around the yeast cells (Fig. 20.1). Specimens of pus, sputum or brain tissue should be digested in KOH and on microscopical examination the resulting cellular debris often delineates the outline of the capsule around the cryptococcal cells.

Dried, heat-fixed and stained smears of clinical material may also be used but it should be noted that processing may cause the collapse of yeast cells to give a crescent-like appearance and these may be difficult to recognize.

In tissue sections, *Cr. neoformans* has a characteristic appearance of round, budding yeast cells surrounded by clear areas denoting the spaces occupied by the capsules (Fig. 20.2). Some of the cells may become distorted during the fixing and embedding procedure and the capsule often shrinks to give the cells a spiny appearance. *Cryptococcus* is difficult to see in HE stained sections and it is best to use a specific fungal stain; alcian blue or mucicarmine, which stain the capsule, are particularly useful. Mucicarmine staining also helps to distinguish *Cryptococcus* from *Histoplasma capsulatum* and *Blastomyces dermatitidis* which either do not stain at all or stain poorly.

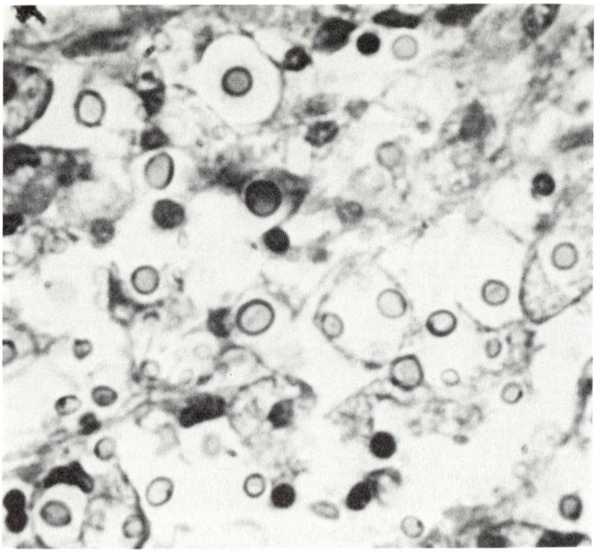

Fig. 20.2 Cryptococcosis. Section of brain showing numerous cells of *Cryptococcus* surrounded by a clear zone which is occupied by capsule (× 400. Stained PAS)

Culture

Clinical material should be cultured on Sabouraud's dextrose, or malt extract agar at 25–37 °C. Cycloheximide, to which *Cr. neoformans* is highly sensitive, should not be used as a supplement. Colonies normally appear within 2–3 days but cultures should be retained for at least 2 weeks before discarding. With c.s.f. a relatively large volume (approx. 5 ml) or a centrifuged deposit should be cultured since the number of cryptococci present varies greatly from one specimen to another and they are often few in number.

Colonies vary from creamy-white and pasty on Sabouraud's dextrose agar to yellow-brown and mucoid on malt extract agar. Identification of isolates depends initially on the recognition of capsules in nigrosine or India ink mounts but it should be remembered that the capsule size will vary according to the medium, incubation temperature and strain of fungus. Capsules are generally narrow on Sabouraud's dextrose agar and at 37 °C but larger on malt extract agar and at lower incubation temperatures (approx. 30 °C).

Cryptococcus species are characterized by their capsule and lack of fermentative ability, and are distinguished from other yeasts with similar features by their ability to produce urease and assimilate inositol. Individual species are identified by their assimilation patterns. *Cr. neoformans* may also be differentiated from other cryptococci by the production of brown pigmented colonies on media containing Niger seed (*Guizotia abyssinica*) extract or caffeic acid (3:4 dihydroxycinnamic acid) and the use of these media for primary isolation enables *Cr. neoformans* colonies to be identified by their pigmentation as soon as they appear.

Animal inoculation

Laboratory animals, with the exception of rabbits, are susceptible to infection with *Cr. neoformans* but animal inoculation is seldom necessary for the purpose of identification of isolates. However, mice may be used if required and intracerebral inoculation will usually cause death within 5–14 days.

Immunology and serology

No satisfactory skin tests are available for cryptococcosis. Serological tests are extremely useful for diagnosis and for establishing the prognosis. Antibodies to *Cr. neoformans* can be detected by IFA and WCA tests but the most useful and the principal diagnostic procedure is the LPA test for the detection of cryptococcal antigen.

Antibody tests

These give positive results in less than 50% of proven cases of cryptococcosis because in patients with active disease an excess of antigen interferes with the demonstration of antibodies. However, antibody tests are of value in detecting early infection and for determining prognosis. The IFA test, which uses heat-killed *Cr. neoformans* cells, has a specificity of around 80% but the WCA test, using formalin-killed cells, is more specific (approx. 95%). The latter also readily allows determination of the antibody titre.

Antigen tests

The antigen detected is the capsular polysaccharide of the yeast which is present throughout the body in patients with active disease. The test is highly sensitive (approx. 92%) and superior to microscopy and culture for the detection of *Cr. neoformans*. False positives are rare. They occur only with specimens of c.s.f. or serum from patients with a high rheumatoid factor titre, although this problem can be overcome by prior treatment of samples with dithiothreitol. A positive result is virtually diagnostic for cryptococcosis.

Antigen detection tests are best done on c.s.f. or serum samples. By diluting the specimen the antigen titre can be determined and this can be directly related to the severity of the infection. The LPA test is most often employed for antigen detection but CIE may also be used and recently ELISA tests have been developed for the detection of both capsular antigen and antibodies.

Serology and prognosis. The progress of the disease can be monitored and decisions made on management by using antigen and antibody tests in combination. In worsening infections the antigen titre rises but successful therapy and remission of the disease results in a decline in antigen titres and the reappearance of antibodies.

TREATMENT

Intravenous amphotericin B in combination with flucytosine is the treatment of choice. Intrathecal amphotericin B may also be used in severe meningeal form. Ketoconazole is under evaluation.

Chapter Twenty-One ASPERGILLOSIS

Aspergillosis, caused most frequently by *Aspergillus fumigatus*, is primarily a pulmonary disease although infections of other sites such as the nasal sinuses and superficial tissues also occur. In its most serious form there is invasion of lung tissues from which dissemination to other organs may follow. More commonly, inhalation of *Aspergillus* spores results in colonization of existing lung cavities (aspergilloma) or a hypersensitivity reaction (allergic aspergillosis).

The spores of aspergilli are ubiquitous in the environment from growth in soil and decaying vegetation.

CLINICAL FORMS

Pulmonary disease

Allergic aspergillosis

Hypersensitivity to aspergilli may manifest as uncomplicated asthma, asthma with pulmonary eosinophilia or extrinsic allergic alveolitis. Uncomplicated asthma (reversible airways obstruction) following inhalation of *Aspergillus* spores is usually seen in atopic individuals who are hypersensitive to a wide range of allergens and have raised IgE levels. Around 10–20% of asthmatics react to *A. fumigatus*. Asthma with eosinophilia of sputum or blood is a more chronic form of the disease and results in progressive lung damage and loss of lung function. It is characterized by episodes of lung consolidation and fleeting shadows on chest X-ray. In the majority (approx. 75%) of these patients the fungus grows in the larger airways to produce plugs of mycelium and mucus which block off segments of lung tissues and even entire lobes; these plugs, which are often coughed up, are a diagnostic feature.

Particularly heavy and repeated exposure to the spores of aspergilli can result in an allergic alveolitis in which the individual suffers breathlessness, fever and malaise some hours after exposure; repeated attacks result in progressive lung damage. A well-known example of this form of aspergillosis is Maltster's lung which occurs in workers who handle barley on which *A. clavatus* has sporulated during the malting process. A survey in Scotland showed that around 5% of malt workers in distilleries had symptoms of this disease.

Aspergilloma

In this form of the disease, also referred to as 'fungus ball', the fungus colonizes pre-existing cavities (often tuberculous) in the lung and forms a compact mass of fungal mycelium which is often surrounded by a dense fibrous wall. Aspergillomas are usually solitary and vary in size ($\leqslant$ 8 cm diam.). Radiologically they have the characteristic appearance of a well-defined mobile opacity within a cavity, usually with a crescent of air at the upper margin.

Patients with an aspergilloma are either symptom-free or have only a moderate degree of cough and sputum production. However, occasional haemoptysis may occur especially when the fungus is actively growing and indeed massive haemorrhage following invasion of a relatively major blood vessel is one of the complications of this condition. Surgical resection is the treatment of choice for most patients but as the prognosis is generally good and symptoms minimal, an aspergilloma can often safely be left untreated and the fungus may die off naturally.

Invasive aspergillosis

Invasive aspergillosis occurs in severely immunocompromised individuals who have serious underlying

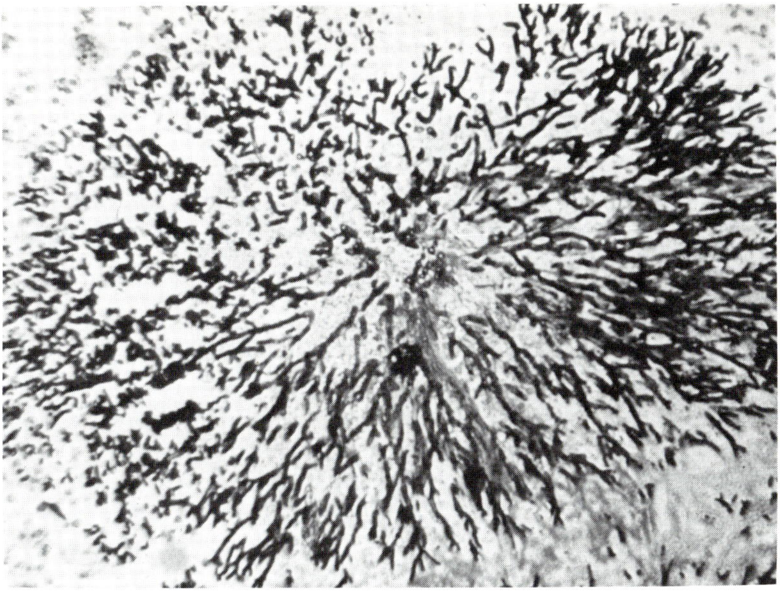

Fig. 21.1 Invasive aspergillosis. Lung section showing spreading, radial growth of *Aspergillus fumigatus* and dichotomous branching of hyphae (× 350. Stained PAS)

illness and/or are receiving cytotoxic or immunosuppressive therapy. Those at risk include individuals with haematological malignancies and transplant patients. A serious reduction in the number of circulating neutrophils (neutropenia) and prior treatment with adrenal corticosteroids are common factors in most of those who develop this form of the disease. There is widespread growth of the fungus in the lung tissue (Fig. 21.1) and the infection may spread from the lungs to involve other organs especially the kidneys and brain.

Invasive aspergillosis has a particularly poor prognosis and is often diagnosed only post-mortem.

Other forms of the disease

Endocarditis

Aspergillus may cause endocarditis in immunosuppressed patients and in those who have undergone open-heart surgery. Clinically, the disease is characterized by large fungal vegetations on the heart valves and a high frequency of emboli. Generally, the condition has a poor prognosis and successful treatment depends on a combination of antifungal therapy and the surgical removal of infected tissue.

Paranasal granuloma

Colonization and invasion of the paranasal sinuses by *A. flavus* and *A. fumigatus* occurs most frequently but not exclusively, among those who live in warm dry climates. The infection may spread through bone to the orbit of the eye and to the brain.

Miscellaneous forms

Aspergillus species may also cause mycotic keratitis and otomycosis (Ch. 10) and onychomycosis (Ch. 9).

EPIDEMIOLOGY

All aspergilli are common saprophytes growing in soil and on decaying plant material. A number of species including *A. fumigatus* are thermophilic so that the biological heating of rotting, composting vegetation promotes their growth and the production of large numbers of spores. Man is constantly exposed to these spores and for those working with decaying vegetation, such as mouldy hay, exposure to counts as high as 21 million spores per cubic metre of air have been recorded. Disease generally follows inhalation of spores but the fungus may also gain entry to the body tissues through wounds or during surgery. Aspergillosis occurs sporadically throughout the world and the frequency with which the various *Aspergillus* species cause disease in different regions may vary with the distribution of the fungi. The prevalent forms of infection also differ, for example, paranasal granuloma caused by *A. flavus* is seen frequently in the Sudan and opportunistic iatrogenic infections caused by *A. fumigatus* occur most often in developed countries where advanced medical procedures involving immunosuppressive drugs and complex surgery are commonly practised.

MYCOLOGY

There are more than 100 species of aspergilli but a

relatively small number have been implicated in human disease. The most important of these are *A. fumigatus*, *A. niger*, *A. flavus*, *A. terreus* and *A. nidulans*. All exist in nature and develop in culture as mycelial fungi and form distinctive sporing structures with thick-walled conidiophores terminating in a vesicle bearing either one or two rows of sterigmata which produce compact chains of conidia. Identification to genus level is relatively simple but the identification of the various species is more difficult and depends mainly on colour and the detailed morphology of the sporing head.

A. fumigatus develops initially as a white colony which becomes grey-green as it sporulates. Conidiophores are approximately 300–500 μm in length, with smooth walls ending in a dome-shaped vesicle. A single row of sterigmata, restricted to the upper-third of the vesicle, produces long chains of roughwalled conidia (2–3.5 μm diam.) (Fig. 21.2). *A. fumigatus*

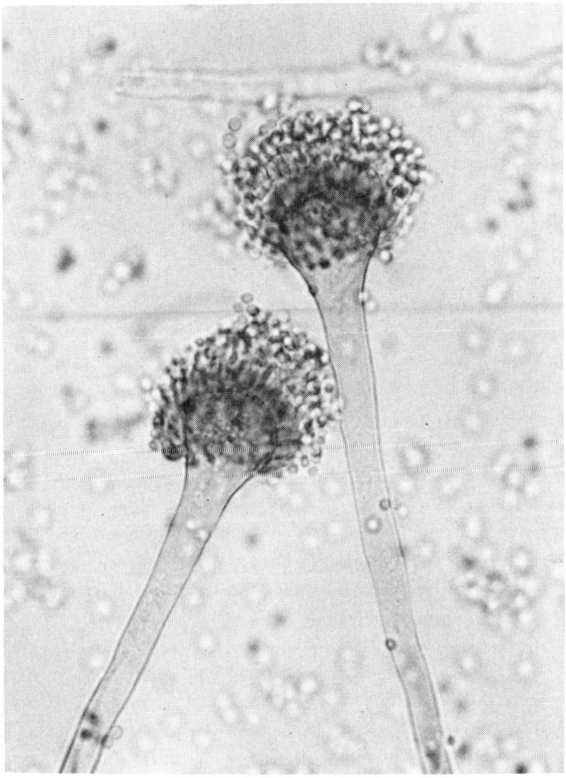

Fig. 21.2 Slide mount of *Aspergillus fumigatus* showing sporing heads (× 550. Cotton Blue/lactophenol)

is markedly thermophilic and will grow at temperatures approaching 50 °C.

DIAGNOSIS

Direct examination

Sputum may be examined in KOH, preferably after digestion with pancreatin, and the fungus appears as septate mycelium with characteristic dichotomous branching (Fig. 21.3).

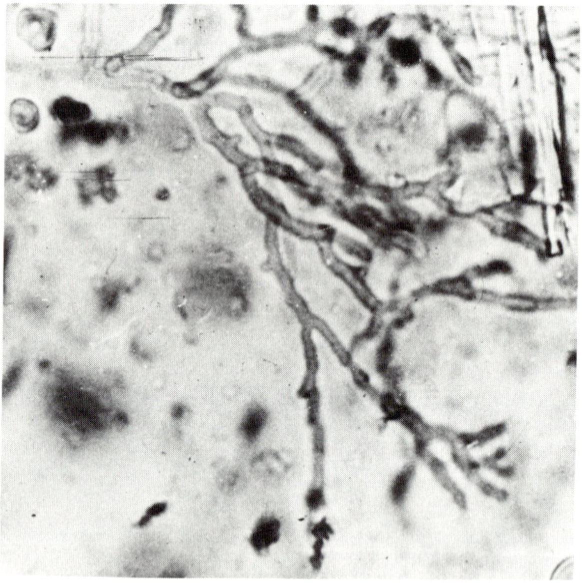

Fig. 21.3 Hyphae of *Aspergillus* in sputum showing characteristic branching and irregular outline (× 400. KOH)

In allergic aspergillosis there is generally an abundance of fungus in the sputum and it is easily detected by microscopy. Moreover, mycelial plugs which may be coughed up are easily recognized with the naked eye. In patients with aspergilloma, fungus may not be consistently seen in sputum and when present it is often in the form of solid wefts of mycelium which have broken free from the fungus ball. In invasive aspergillosis microscopy is often negative and in patients with suspected invasive disease, biopsy may be the only method of making a definitive diagnosis.

In tissue, *Aspergillus* produces non-pigmented

septate hyphae (3–5 μm diam.) which characteristically show repeated dichotomous branching and have an irregular outline. On rare occasions when the fungus is growing in an open airway the characteristic sporing heads may be produced. HE staining is of little value and the fungus is best seen in tissue sections stained with PAS, methenamine-silver or Gridley stains.

Culture

Aspergilli grow readily in culture on routine media such as Sabouraud's dextrose agar at 25–37 °C and colonies appear after 24–48 hours' incubation. The ability of *A. fumigatus* to grow well at 45 °C can be used as an aid to the identification of this species.

Sputum should preferably be cultured quantitatively. The sputum is digested in pancreatin, centrifuged, the supernatant discarded and the debris resuspended in saline to the original volume; a measured aliquot of this is cultured and the results used to calculate the number of colony forming units (c.f.u.) per ml of sputum. As aspergilli are ubiquitous, quantitative assessments of the amount of fungus in sputum help confirm that a positive culture is not due to chance contamination and is also useful for monitoring the progress of the disease and the response to therapy.

Culture results mimic those for direct microscopy in that large amounts of fungus are usually recovered from the sputum of patients with allergic aspergillosis but cultures from patients with aspergilloma or invasive disease may be negative or yield only a few colonies. In invasive aspergillosis blood cultures are usually negative and examination of biopsy material is necessary for diagnosis.

Animal inoculation

This is neither useful nor necessary for diagnosis of the disease or the identification of aspergilli.

Immunology and serology

Skin tests

Skin tests with *A. fumigatus* antigen are useful in the

diagnosis of allergic aspergillosis. Patients with uncomplicated asthma due to aspergilli give an immediate type I reaction. Those with asthma and pulmonary eosinophilia give an immediate type I reaction and 70% also give a delayed type III arthus reaction. Specific IgE antibodies to aspergilli can also be detected in these patients using radioallergosorbent (RAST) tests.

Skin test results are variable in patients with extrinsic allergic alveolitis and are generally not of diagnostic value.

Serological tests

Tests (ID and CIE) for the detection of precipitins to *Aspergillus* (IgG antibodies) are widely used for the diagnosis of all forms of aspergillosis. Culture filtrate and somatic antigens of *A. fumigatus*, *A. niger* and *A. flavus* are used routinely, although many laboratories use only *A. fumigatus* extracts, relying on cross-reactivity between the antigens of this species and those of the other pathogenic aspergilli.

Low levels of precipitating antibodies to *Aspergillus* can be detected in 60–70% of patients with allergic aspergillosis and eosinophilia but after concentration of sera the proportion rises to around 90%; typically only one or two precipitin lines develop in ID or CIE tests. Patients with extrinsic allergic alveolitis due to *Aspergillus* also develop precipitating antibodies.

In aspergilloma there is a strong precipitin response because of the more prolonged exposure to the fungus (Fig. 21.4). The precipitin test is positive in over 90% of patients with aspergilloma and almost 80% have 6 or more precipitin lines on ID or CIE. A strongly positive precipitin test to *Aspergillus* together with the characteristic radiological picture is diagnostic for aspergilloma.

When clinical and radiological evidence suggests an aspergilloma but the precipitin test with *A. fumigatus* is negative or weakly positive then the possibility that another species of *Aspergillus* or another pathogenic fungus such as *Pseudallescheria* (*Petriellidium*) *boydii* is responsible should be considered.

In invasive aspergillosis, although precipitins may be produced, they are seldom present in quantity

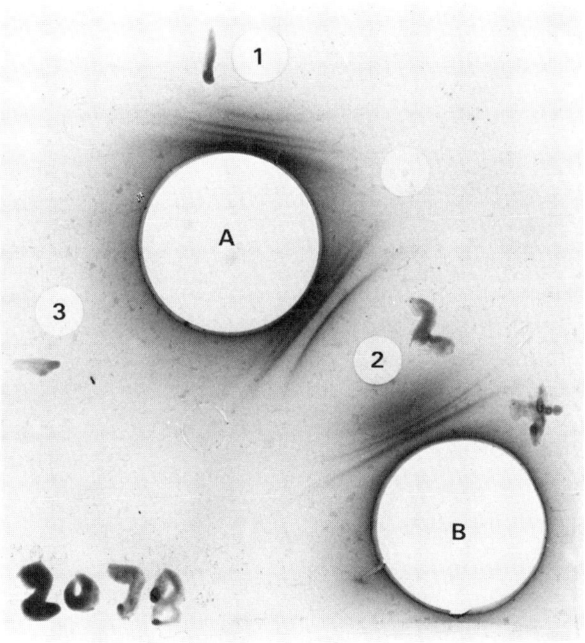

Fig. 21.4 Immunodiffusion plate showing strong precipitin reaction in serum of patient with aspergilloma (Stained Coomassie Blue BL). Key to wells: A. patient's serum; B. positive control serum; 1. *Aspergillus fumigatus* culture filtrate antigens; 2. *A. fumigatus* somatic antigens; 3. negative control (saline)

because of impaired immunity caused by the patient's underlying illness or chemotherapy; in some instances patients may die without producing detectable antibodies.

Patients with *Aspergillus* endocarditis usually have demonstrable precipitins and this can be very helpful in establishing the diagnosis.

Antibody titres decrease on successful therapy or for instance after surgical removal of an aspergilloma and can be used to confirm successful treatment.

CF, IFA and PHA tests for the detection of antibodies to *Aspergillus* have also been reported but at present these tests are not widely used.

Antigen detection. Tests for the detection of circulating *Aspergillus* antigen based on CIE, RIA and ELISA have recently been described for use in patients with invasive disease — these are of particular value for early diagnosis of infection and for use in patients who fail to produce demonstrable antibodies to *Aspergillus*.

TREATMENT

Allergic. Corticosteroids.

Aspergilloma. Surgical excision or conservative management.

Invasive. Intravenous amphotericin B. Concomitant flucytosine may help. Reduce immunosuppression when possible.

Chapter Twenty-Two SYSTEMIC CANDIDOSIS

(Synonym: systemic candidiasis)

Systemic forms of candidosis, caused by members of the genus *Candida*, may be localized in one or more organs, such as the urinary tract, heart valves (endocarditis) and meninges or may be widely disseminated and associated with a yeast septicaemia (candidaemia). Disease results from the development of commensal organisms associated with some serious localized or general abnormality of the host. Although systemic candidosis occurs much less frequently than the superficial forms of this disease (Ch. 7) the incidence of these often iatrogenic infections has increased during recent years with the advent of advanced medical and surgical treatments. Deep-seated candidosis is difficult to diagnose and prognosis is generally poor.

CLINICAL FORMS

Candidaemia occurs mainly in postoperative or immunosuppressed patients and the main clinical sign is an intermittent elevated temperature. In some patients the candidaemia is transient and may clear spontaneously, in others it is associated with the presence of contaminated intravenous catheters and disappears when these are removed. However, a proportion of patients with candidaemia go on to develop generalized or localized infection.

One common clinical sign of deep tissue invasion is the appearance of white candidal lesions within the eye (*Candida* endophthalmitis). Common sites of involvement in disseminated infection include the kidney, for which *C. albicans* has a recognized predilection, the brain and the gastrointestinal tract. The heart may also be a focus of infection following bloodborne spread of *Candida* but the majority of cases of *Candida* endocarditis follow surgery for valve replacement. The mitral and aortic valves are usually involved and characteristically there are large fungal vegetations which are friable and frequently cause emboli in the major arteries. Yeast endocarditis is also a recognized hazard for drug addicts who inject themselves with contaminated material and the disease may also occasionally be seen in patients on immunosuppressive therapy.

Urinary tract infections due to *Candida* may affect the kidneys or may be localized in the bladder or, on rare occasions, in the urethra. Infection of the kidney is usually bloodborne but ascending infection can also occur. In most cases urinary infections are associated either with the presence of an indwelling bladder catheter, previous disease or surgery of the urinary tract, urinary stasis, diabetes mellitus or treatment with antibiotics. The infection often clears when the underlying cause is corrected.

Occasionally a superficial infection of the mouth may spread to involve other parts of the alimentary tract, notably the oesophagus and this is a well-recognized complication in leukaemic patients. *Candida* infection may also spread from the mouth to the lungs where it involves the main bronchi and on rarer occasions the parenchyma of the lung.

EPIDEMIOLOGY

The source of infection in systemic candidosis is the same as for superficial forms of the disease, namely commensal *Candida* species. The opportunity for endogenous infection is greatest among hospitalized patients in whom the carriage rate of yeasts in the mouth and gastrointestinal tract is known to be higher than that of the normal population. For example, surveys have shown a frequency of yeasts in the mouth ranging from 13–76% for hospital patients compared to 2–37% in normal individuals.

Numerous factors are known to predispose to yeast overgrowth (see Table 7.1) but the highest numbers of yeasts occur in patients treated with antibiotics or steroids, in poorly controlled diabetics and after surgical procedures such as transplant or heart surgery which involve complex supportive therapy. In such patients *Candida* may enter the deep tissues via the respiratory or urinary tracts or when intravenous catheters, wound or operation sites become contaminated. Most often, however, entry is through the gastrointestinal tract where the organism passes across intact intestinal mucosa into the bloodstream by a process of persorption. This intrusion of yeasts into the bloodstream is known to occur relatively frequently but is most often transient in nature and clearly it is abnormalities of the host rather than the entry of the fungus which is of greatest importance in establishment of infection.

Systemic candidosis occurs rarely and usually only in those in which an underlying disease and/or its treatment predisposes them to yeast overgrowth and at the same time severely impairs their resistance to infection (see Table 7.1).

MYCOLOGY

Mycological aspects are as outlined in Chapter 7 on superficial candidosis. *C. albicans* accounts for the majority of systemic infections but *C. tropicalis* is also frequently implicated and *C. parapsilosis* is responsible for some 25% of yeast endocarditis. *C. glabrata* is frequently involved in infections of the urinary tract.

DIAGNOSIS

Diagnosis of the deep-seated forms of candidosis presents considerable difficulties. Clinically there is usually little to suggest that a deep infection is due to *Candida* except when lesions of the eye (endophthalmitis) are noted. Laboratory tests frequently give equivocal results because of the commensal status of *Candida*. The isolation of *Candida* from clinical material, except from sites that are normally sterile, is of little significance and it is difficult also to attach any value to the numbers of yeasts isolated since these may be considerable in the absence of infection. A similar problem occurs with serology since antibodies to *Candida* can be detected in uninfected individuals because of their exposure to commensal yeasts.

In general, a series of tests is more useful than a single investigation since it is the changes in the number of yeasts present or in the antibody titre which is of greatest diagnostic significance. The results of culture and serology must therefore be interpreted subjectively together with the clinical findings and efforts should be made to obtain biopsy material to examine for evidence of tissue invasion.

Direct examination

In suspected systemic infection samples of sputum, urine, c.s.f., etc. may be examined microscopically in KOH or after Gram staining. In tissue sections the fungus is best seen if stained with PAS or methenamine-silver stains (Fig. 22.1). Mycelium is particularly abundant in tissue from deep-seated infection

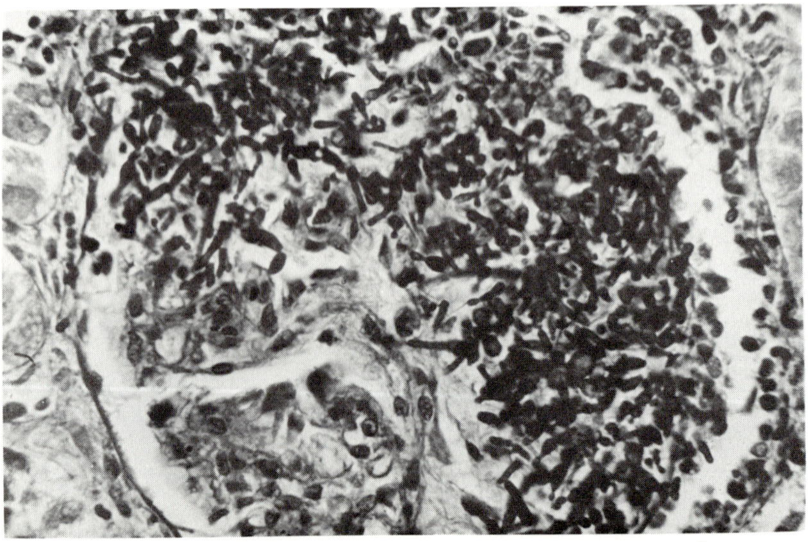

Fig. 22.1 Systemic candidosis. Section of kidney showing mass of hyphae and yeast cells of *Candida albicans* in glomerulus (× 350. Stained PAS)

but, contrary to the commonly held belief, the presence of *Candida* mycelium in sputum or urine samples does not confirm that the yeast is present as a pathogen.

Culture

Candida spp. are easily recovered from clinical material in culture at 37°C on common isolation media (Ch. 7). In cases of suspected systemic candidosis cultures should be made from as many sources as possible and efforts should also be made to obtain material suitable for direct examination. Blood cultures, taken into vented culture bottles, provide the most reliable evidence of systemic infection although repeated attempts to isolate the organism may be necessary, particularly in patients with *Candida* endocarditis. Although isolation of *Candida* from the bloodstream should always be taken seriously and further investigations made immediately, it must nevertheless be borne in mind that candidaemias which are transient and of no clinical significance do occur. Isolation from peritoneal fluid and c.s.f. provides reliable evidence for the diagnosis of *Candida* peritonitis (which occurs most often in patients on peritoneal dialysis) and *Candida* meningitis respectively. Cultures obtained from urine, faeces and sputum are of little diagnostic value since they are positive in a large proportion of hospitalized patients and investigation of these samples is usually only of value if done quantitatively over a period of time. Counts of *Candida* in the urine in excess of 10^4 per ml are usually taken to indicate urinary tract infection except in patients with indwelling urinary catheters. Yeasts are usually present in the urine of patients with systemic candidosis but a positive urine culture does not confirm systemic involvement. Particular care must be taken in interpreting the results of sputum cultures as sputum is frequently contaminated with *Candida* from the mouth. Culture of bronchial secretions provides more reliable evidence of lung colonization or infection.

Since *Candida* multiplies rapidly in clinical material such as sputum or urine, it is important that specimens are processed immediately after collection.

Animal inoculation

Although laboratory animals such as rabbits and mice are susceptible to infection with *Candida*, animal inoculation is neither useful nor necessary for identification of isolates or for confirmation of pathogenicity.

Immunology and serology

Skin tests

Skin testing is of no diagnostic value as the majority of the population give a positive reaction.

Serological tests

These are useful in the diagnosis of deep-seated candidosis although they lack sensitivity and specificity and the results must be interpreted with care. The most widely used tests are WCA using killed *Candida* cells and ID or CIE for the detection of precipitins to cytoplasmic extracts of *Candida*. It is recommended that both the agglutinin and precipitin tests are carried out using antigens from more than one species but in practice it is usually adequate to use *C. albicans* and *C.parapsilosis* antigens since these species virtually cover the spectrum of antigens found among the potentially pathogenic members of the genus.

A positive test does not necessarily indicate infection since both agglutinins and precipitins are widespread among individuals who have no obvious *Candida* infection. These are undoubtedly produced in response to high levels of commensal yeasts and it has been shown that the antibody titre fluctuates with changes in their numbers. However, most of those who harbour large numbers of commensal *Candida* do so for a short time only and the titre declines as the flora returns to normal; this serves to distinguish them from infected individuals, in whom the antibody titre remains elevated or continues to rise.

It is considered that the cell wall mannan, which inevitably contaminates somatic extracts of *Candida*, is the component in the antigen which is responsible for the majority of the positive precipitin reactions seen in uninfected individuals. Reactions to the protein/glycoprotein components of the extract, on the other hand, are known to occur mainly in those with systemic infection and consequently are of greater diagnostic significance. The type of precipitin reaction must therefore be taken into account; precipitin lines to mannan are broad and fuzzy and are usually easily distinguished from the thin, sharply defined protein/glycoprotein lines. If possible an extract from which the mannan has been removed by affinity chromatography with Concanavalin A sepharose should be used for diagnostic testing.

A negative antibody test does not necessarily rule out the possibility of deep-seated candidosis since a significant proportion of those who become systemically infected with *Candida* are immunologically compromised and incapable of mounting a detectable antibody response.

Other serological tests such as LPA, IFA and PHA are also available for diagnosis of systemic candidosis but they suffer the same drawbacks as the agglutination and precipitin tests and often to a greater extent. ELISA tests for the detection of *Candida* antibodies offer a much improved sensitivity but their diagnostic potential is still being evaluated.

Despite their limitations serological tests are of diagnostic value when used sensibly. They are most useful when a series of tests is performed at regular intervals over a period of time; a high or rapidly rising antibody titre suggests infection and conversely a reduction in titre indicates recovery from the disease.

Antigen detection. Tests for antigen have recently been introduced for the diagnosis of *Candida* infections and these are of particular value in patients who fail to produce antibodies. The various methods, for example ELISA, RIA and PHA, which detect either cell wall mannan or cytoplasmic components require further refinement and improvement in sensitivity. However, the results obtained so far have been sufficiently encouraging to suggest that antigen detection will eventually become the principal method for serodiagnosis of systemic candidosis.

TREATMENT

Intravenous amphotericin B, sometimes in combination with flucytosine. Flucytosine may be used alone in candiduria providing the isolate is sensitive. Oral ketoconazole has been used successfully. Surgery is generally also required in endocarditis.

Chapter Twenty-Three
PHYCOMYCOSIS

(Synonyms: zygomycosis; mucormycosis)

Phycomycosis is used as a general term for a group of infections caused by a number of lower fungi. Although the various fungi have a common tissue form of broad, aseptate hyphae the type of disease differs according to the causal fungus. More specific nomenclature is used for the different clinical forms.

CLINICAL FORMS

Rhinocerebral disease

Rhinocerebral infection may be caused by a number of different fungi, most commonly species of *Mucor, Absidia* and *Rhizopus* and this form of the disease is also referred to as mucormycosis. It is the most serious and rapidly fulminating form of phycomycosis and is almost invariably associated either with acute diabetes mellitus and ketoacidosis or with debilitating diseases such as leukaemia or lymphoma. It results in extensive and rapid destruction of tissues, most commonly spreading from the nasal mucosa to the turbinate bone, paranasal sinuses, orbit and brain where massive invasion of blood vessels causes major infarcts (Fig. 23.1). Spread may also occur to the lungs, gastrointestinal tract, skin and occasionally to other organs.

The same group of fungi may also cause pulmonary or systemic infection without rhinocerebral involvement, usually in severely immunocompromised individuals, especially those with leukaemia. Primary cutaneous infections have also been reported but these are extremely rare and usually occur in patients with severe burns. Rhinocerebral phycomycosis is usually fatal and many diagnoses are made only at necropsy.

Subcutaneous disease

There are two distinct forms of subcutaneous disease depending on which of two closely related species of fungi is involved.

Basidiobolomycosis

In this disease caused by *Basidiobolus haptosporus*, infection develops to form a well circumscribed, firm but painless subcutaneous nodule and slowly progresses to form a large mass which is attached to the skin but moves freely over the underlying muscle. Involvement of the underlying tissues is rare. The limbs and buttocks are most frequently involved but any part of the body may be affected and extensive, grossly swollen areas may develop.

Entomophthoromycosis

The causal fungus is *Conidiobolus coronatus*, previously known as *Entomophthora coronata*. The infection, which is also referred to as rhinoentomophthoromycosis, orginates usually in the nasal mucosa and spreads to the nasal sinuses and adjacent subcutaneous tissues of the face. Characteristically, nasal polyps develop and there is gross facial swelling, although there is little or no pain. Unlike basidiobolomycosis the lesions are firmly attached to the underlying tissues.

Both forms of subcutaneous phycomycosis generally remain localized and are rarely fatal.

EPIDEMIOLOGY

All forms of phycomycosis occur following exposure to the causal fungi living as saprophytes in the environment.

The causal agents of rhinocerebral phycomycosis, commonly referred to as 'bread moulds' or 'pin moulds', occur on a wide range of substrates including soil. Sporadic infections occur throughout the world but the virulence of these fungi is clearly of a low order and despite their ubiquitous nature, rhinocerebral phycomycosis occurs only rarely and in severely debilitated individuals.

There is no evidence to suggest that subcutaneous forms of phycomycosis are confined to the debilitated or those with impaired immunity. The distribution of infections is, nevertheless, more restricted than the distribution of the causal fungi. *C. coronatus* is found on decaying vegetation in most warm climates but infections, which occur mainly in adult males, predominate among those living or working in the tropical rain forests of Africa, South and Central America and South East Asia. *B. haptosporus* also occurs on decaying plant material in tropical and subtropical regions. It is commonly found also in the gastrointestinal tract of amphibians and small reptiles but whether this has any epidemiological significance is uncertain. Infections occur mainly in children and young adults, usually males, and the majority of diagnosed cases have occurred in Indonesia and other tropical parts of South-East Asia and in Africa.

MYCOLOGY

The causal agents of the various forms of phycomycosis are classified within the Zygomycotina, Class Zygomycetes. Those that cause rhinocerebral phycomycosis belong to the Order Mucorales and are characterized by the production of asexual spores enclosed within a sporangium. Colonies are usually fast growing, off-white to pale grey in colour and deeply floccose. Sexual reproduction with zygospore formation is rarely seen in clinical isolates.

Conidiobolus and *Basidiobolus* belong to the Order Entomophthorales. Mature colonies of both fungi are pale grey or buff coloured and compact, folded and waxy in appearance. Asexual reproduction occurs by the formation of detachable multinucleate sporangia (also loosely termed conidia) on distinctively shaped sporangiophores. The sporangia are forcibly discharged which results in a visible film of spores being formed on test-tube walls or on the lids of petri-dishes when these fungi are cultured. The hyphae of *Conidiobolus* and *Basidiobolus* have occasional septa. In *Basidiobolus* both chlamydospores and zygospores are regularly formed. Zygospores are rarely produced in *Conidiobolus* cultures but chlamydospores are common.

DIAGNOSIS

Laboratory diagnosis of rhinocerebral phycomycosis is difficult because of the rapid fulminating course of the disease and because of the doubtful significance of isolates of fungi which are commonly encountered as laboratory contaminants. Recognition of the fungus in tissue by microscopy is considerably more reliable than culture (Fig. 23.1) but material such as nasal discharge or sputum seldom contains much fungal material and examination of a biopsy is usually necessary for firm diagnosis.

Subcutaneous forms of phycomycosis are seldom fatal and the need for a rapid diagnosis is less urgent.

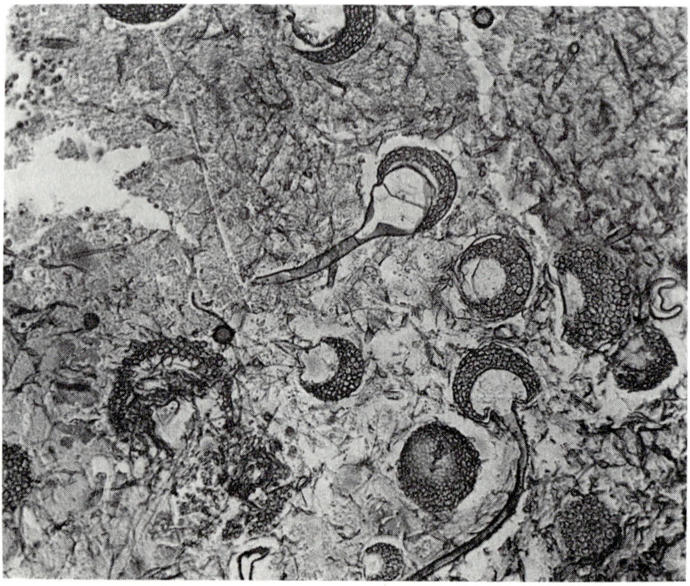

Fig. 23.1 Rhinocerebral phycomycosis due to *Rhizopus sp*. Relatively unusual finding of sporangia in section of mid-turbinate bone (× 120. Stained HE)

Biopsy material is again the most suitable for investigation, and here culture and direct examination are equally helpful.

Direct examination

Microscopical examination of curetted or biopsy material and discharges digested in KOH may reveal the characteristic broad, aseptate, branched and sometimes distorted hyphae. However, these are usually only very sparsely distributed through the infected tissue (Fig. 23.2) and a staining procedure should be used whenever possible. Although the hyphae may be detected in HE stained sections, they are seen much more clearly when stained with methenamine silver. The hyphae of these fungi do not stain with PAS.

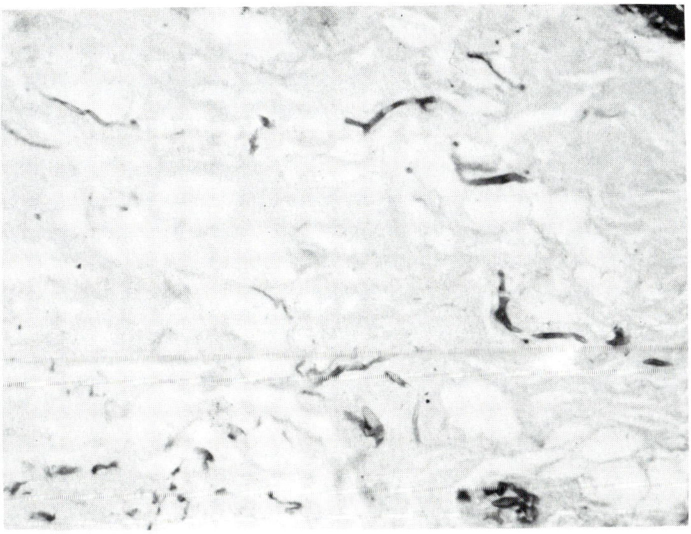

Fig. 23.2 Basidiobolomycosis. Section showing sparse, branched aseptate hyphae of *Basidiobolus haptosporus*. Infection of buttock in child in India (× 80. Stained HE)

Culture

The causal fungi are readily isolated on Sabouraud's dextrose agar containing an antibacterial supplement at 37 °C. The isolation of *Basidiobolus* or *Conidiobolus* is virtually diagnostic but the isolation of species of Mucorales is usually of little significance and requires confirmation by direct examination or strong supporting clinical evidence.

Animal inoculation

Conidiobolus infections in horses and infections with mucoraceous fungi in various wild and domestic animals have been recorded. However, the inoculation of animals with clinical isolates of these fungi is no diagnostic value.

Serology

There are at present no satisfactory serological procedures to assist in the diagnosis of any of the forms of phycomycosis.

TREATMENT

Subcutaneous forms. Long term therapy with potassium iodide and cotrimoxazole. Intravenous amphotericin B if this fails.

Other forms. Intravenous amphotericin B.

APPENDIX

EXAMINATION OF FUNGI

Preparation of wet slide mounts for microscopy

Material from cultures should be taken by stiff inoculating wire with its end bent to form a right-angled hook rather than a loop. If the growth is compact (powdery, velvety or granular) it may be helpful to take a little of the agar medium together with the fungus. The material should be disturbed as little as possible during transfer but, if necessary, it may be teased out very gently on the slide. Examination should first of all be made using the low power (×10) objective, switching to high power (×40) only for more detailed examination of regions which seem likely to give the information required or to obtain detail of small spores etc. The oil immersion (×100) objective is only rarely required. It will be found that the thinner parts, usually around the edges of the mounted material, give the best results. More than one mount may be necessary and parts of the colony showing different texture or colour should also be examined.

The procedure is as follows:

1. Immerse fungal material in a drop of 95% alcohol, previously placed on the slide, to drive out the air trapped within and between the hyphae. Add the mountant before the alcohol dries out.

2. Use 1, or at the most 2 drops of mountant. (A common fault is to add too much.)

3. Touch one edge of the drop of mountant with the cover-glass edge and lower gently, avoiding air bubbles.

In addition to the examination of slide mounts it is often useful to study fungal growth in situ and this can be done under a low power (×2.5; ×10) objective, either using petri-dish cultures or the edges of slope cultures where the growth impinges on the glass wall of the test-tube. (Care must be taken to distinguish globules of water from fungal structures such as sporangia.)

Slide culture

This technique, which allows fungal growth to be examined undisturbed, depends on the hyphae and sporophores attaching themselves to glass. The coverglass and slide used in the technique must therefore be free from grease and the humidity of culture vessel must be maintained. Best results are obtained with fungi without organized sporophores (i.e. when spores are produced on vegetative hyphae as, for example, in dermatophytes). Slide culture is therefore not suitable for all fungi.

The method is as follows:

1 Flame sterilize slides and place on bent glass rod supports in petri-dishes.

2. Prepare a petri-dish of medium suitable for growth of the fungus under investigation.

3. With sterile needle or small scalpel blade cut solidified medium into squares of approximately 0.75–1.0 cm.

4. Aseptically transfer a square of agar to the centre of slide within petri-dish and inoculate each edge of the square with fungus.

5. Remove coverglass which has been immersed in alcohol with forceps, touch on bunsen flame and place on top of inoculated agar square.

6. Add sterile water to base of petri-dish, ensuring it does not touch slide, and incubate. Duration of incubation varies with the species of fungus. Decide when the culture is ready for mounting according to amount of growth visible to the eye or by microscopical examination of the preparation either directly

within the petri-dish or by removing the slide to a microscope stage.

7. When sufficient growth has occurred, remove coverglass and place with growth upwards on clean slide. Add drop of 95% alcohol to centre and allow to spread outwards to drive air from fungal growth — add a drop of mountant and mount on slide. (A second preparation can usually be prepared from the slide, the agar block being removed and disposed of in a disinfectant jar.)

Permanent preparations

Mounts in lactophenol or similar mountant will usually keep for several weeks. If it is desired to retain preparations for longer periods the edges of the coverglass should be sealed off to prevent drying out. There are a number of commercially available sealants (e.g. Aquaseel, Raymond A. Lamb, London) but nail varnish gives good results. In all cases excess mountant should be removed to give a dry, clean surface at junction of the slide and coverglass. Properly sealed, the preparations can be kept for many years.

MOUNTANTS

Lactophenol

Phenol crystals 20 g; lactic acid 20 ml; glycerol 40 ml; distilled H_2O 20 ml. Heat gently to dissolve. Keep in a dark bottle away from direct light. Lactophenol which is a clearing agent may be used alone for preparation of slide mounts but it is usual to add a dye.

Lactophenol Cotton Blue

Lactophenol 100 ml; Cotton Blue 0.075 g (Raymond A. Lamb, London; BDH Chemicals, Poole). Allow to stand for a few days and filter. Available ready made from BDH Chemicals, Poole.

Lactic acid and Cotton Blue

Lactic acid is used in place of lactophenol.

Light Green

Quantities and preparation as for Cotton blue but using Light Green SF (Raymond A. Lamb, London; BDH Chemicals, Poole).

The Cotton Blue mountants stain the fungal hyphae, particularly the young growing parts with dense cytoplasmic contents, a deep blue. The intensity of staining increases with time and may blot out certain aspects of morphology. If Light Green is used the staining is less intense and mounts can be kept for long periods without losing detail of structure.

IDENTIFICATION OF YEASTS

Because of their limited range of morphological features, biochemical criteria have largely replaced morphology as the basis for identification of yeasts. The methods are outlined below but for full details reference should be made to more comprehensive texts.

Kits for identification of medically important yeasts are available commercially, for example, from API (API System S.A., Montalieu-Vercieu, France).

Fermentation of sugars/assimilation of carbon and nitrogen compounds

In the case of fermentation tests a positive result is recorded when there is both acid and gas production; acid production alone is too variable a criterion for identification purposes since different isolates of the same species frequently give variable results. Assimilation tests may be carried out in liquid media containing a single source of carbon or nitrogen, or by the auxanographic method. With the auxanographic method, molten cooled agar which lacks either a carbon or nitrogen source, is seeded with the yeast and poured into a petri-dish, allowed to solidify and paper discs impregnated with different carbon or nitrogen sources are placed on the agar surface — growth of the yeast around individual discs indicates assimilation of that particular compound.

The assimilation and fermentation pattern is used to identify the isolate.

Mycelium/pseudomycelium production

The ability of the yeast to form mycelium/ pseudomycelium is tested using the following procedure:

1. Melt a universal container of potato-dextrose agar and pour into a sterile petri-dish. Coat a sterile glass slide by immersing in the molten agar. Place on the glass rod support in a petri-dish to allow the coating of agar to solidify.
2. Remove a light inoculum from a culture of the yeast to be investigated and streak lightly along the length of the agar on the upper surface of the slide.
3. Place a sterile coverglass over the centre of the inoculated agar. Pour a few millilitres of sterile water into the base of the slide culture dish (to prevent the agar drying out) and incubate at 28 °C.
4. After 2–3 days remove from the incubator, wipe agar from underside of slide, examine microscopically for presence or absence of pseudomycelium or true mycelium.

Rapid identification of Candida albicans

1. Chlamydospore production

Prepare a petri-dish of Czapek Dox+Tween 80 agar. Take a light inoculum from the yeast culture and, taking a centre line in the dish, cut across and through the agar to the dish base. Lift the agar on both sides of the streak with the inoculating wire and allow the inoculum to spread between the lower surface of the agar and the dish. Incubate at 28 °C. After 24 hours examine from the reverse side of the dish under the low (×10) power of the microscope.

If round, thick-walled chlamydospores are produced the yeast is *C. albicans* (Fig. 7.4b).

2. Germ tube production in serum

Place 0.5ml amounts of human or horse serum in small test-tubes and inoculate with a loopful of the yeast to be tested. Incubate at 37 °C, preferably in a water bath, for $1\frac{1}{2}$–2 h. Remove a drop of serum to a slide, add a coverslip and examine microscopically for germ tube production. If germ tubes are produced within this period, giving the cells a drumstick appearance, the yeast is *C. albicans* (Fig. 7.4a).

MEDIA

Many media are available commercially in dehydrated form. There are a number of manufacturers but Difco Laboratories (Detroit, Michigan) and Oxoid Ltd (Basingstoke) produce a wide range of mycological media.

For isolation of fungi from clinical material the media may be supplemented with antibacterial antibiotics, usually chloramphenicol, and with cycloheximide to control contamination with bacteria and saprophytic fungi respectively (see later). After distribution, media are autoclaved at 121°C for 15 minutes, unless otherwise stated.

General purpose media

Malt extract agar

Malt extract* 20 or 40 g; agar 20 g; distilled H_2O 1000 ml. A 3% malt extract agar is available commercially from a variety of sources and is a suitable substitute for 4%. The 2% medium is satisfactory for the isolation, growth and conservation of most fungi. 4% medium is used for the isolation of dermatophytes and other pathogenic fungi (not aspergilli).

Sabouraud's dextrose agar (glucose-peptone agar)

Dextrose 40 g; peptone (mycological) 10 g; agar 20 g; distilled H_2O 1000ml.

This medium is used for isolation and culture of dermatophytes and other pathogenic fungi requiring a rich substrate with a high content of organic nitrogen. Available commercially from a variety of sources, although the type of peptone may vary according to the manufacturer.

* Source in UK, Boots Pure Drug Co., Nottingham. Properties of malt extract may vary from batch to batch and according to the manufacturer but all are satisfactory for use as isolation media.

Czapek-Dox agar

$MgSO_4$ 0.5 g; KCl 0.5 g; $NaNO_3$ 2.0 g; $FeSO_4$ 0.01 g; K_2HPO_4 1.0 g; sucrose 30.0 g; agar 20.0 g.

Czapek-Dox medium is recommended for culture of the penicillia and aspergilli. It is satisfactory for most saprophytes except the Zygomycetes which do better on 2% malt extract. Can be used to differentiate dermatophytes from saprophytes; the former do not grow on this medium.

Special media for dermatophytes

Nutrient agar

Beef extract (Lab Lemco) 10 g; Peptone (Oxoid, bacteriological) 10 g; NaCl 5g; agar 20 g; distilled H_2O 1000 ml.

Preferred to Sabouraud's dextrose or malt extract agar for the isolation of *Trichophyton verrucosum*.

Urea agar

Urea agar base (Oxoid) 2.4 g; distilled H_2O 95 ml. Boil to dissolve the agar and autoclave at 115°C for 20 min. Cool to 55°C and aseptically add 5 ml sterile 40% urea solution and distribute.

Used to differentiate between *T. rubrum* and *T. mentagrophytes*; the urease activity of *T. mentagrophytes* turns the indicator in the medium red within 2–3 days whereas *T. rubrum* either does not produce urease, or takes much longer to do so.

Yeast identification media

Sugar fermentation medium

Peptone water (Oxoid) 15 g; Andrades Indicator* 10 ml; distilled H_2O 1000 ml.

Sugar is added to a concentration of 3% (w/v) and distributed in 3 ml quantities into 10 × 1 cm tubes containing an inverted Durham tube. Either sterilize in a Koch sterilizer for 30 min on 3 consecutive days

* *Andrades Indicator* — acid fuchsin 0.5% in distilled H_2O. Add 1N-NaOH until colour just turns yellow. Phenol red may be used as an alternative indicator.

— the gas trapped in the Durham tube is driven out during the process — or filter sterilize.

Assimilation test media

Auxanographic procedure

1. Yeast-nitrogen base (carbon free). KH_2PO_4 1.0 g; $MgSO_4$ 0.5 g; $(NH_4)_2SO_4$ 5.0 g; agar 25.0 g; distilled H_2O 1000 ml.

Dissolve ingredients in distilled water, boiling to melt agar; dispense 20 ml lots into universal containers and autoclave at 115°C for 15 min.

Available from Difco. Convenient to make up at 10 × strength, filter sterilize and add to sterile agar solution to dilute.

2. Yeast carbon base (nitrogen free). KH_2PO_4 1.0g; $MgSO_4$ 0.5 g; dextrose 20.0 g; agar 25.0 g; distilled H_2O 1000 ml.

Preparation is as for carbon free base.

Available from Difco. Make up as before.

Sugar impregnated discs (for use with yeast nitrogen base)

Lay out 5 mm diameter filter paper discs on glass sheets and pipette a drop of saturated sugar solution onto each disc. Remove any excess solution with a Pasteur pipette and allow the discs to dry at 37°C. Alternatively discs may be freeze-dried.

Peptone/KNO_3 impregnated discs (for use with yeast carbon base)

Prepare as for sugar discs.

It is useful to use different coloured filter paper discs so that individual substrates may be easily identified.

Potato-dextrose agar

Potato-dextrose agar (Oxoid) 39 g; distilled H_2O 1000 ml. Boil to melt agar, distribute into universal containers and autoclave.

Used for production of mycelium/pseudomycelium by yeasts.

Czapek Dox+Tween 80 agar

Czapek Dox agar (modified) Oxoid 45.4 g; Tween 80 10 ml; distilled H_2O 1000 ml.

Boil to melt agar, distribute into universal containers and autoclave.

Used to test for chlamydospore production by *Candida albicans* and also for the production of mycelium/pseudomycelium by yeasts.

Urea agar

(See p. 181) Used to test for urease production — a feature of *Cryptococcus* spp.

Niger seed (Guizotia abyssinica) medium

Dextrose 10.0 g; creatinine 0.78 g; *Guizotia abyssinica* extract* 200 ml; agar 20.0 g; distilled H_2O 800 ml.

Caffeic acid medium

Dextrose 5.0 g; $(NH_4)_2SO_4$ 5.0 g; yeast extract 2.0 g; KH_2PO_4 0.8 g; $MgSO_4$ 0.7 g; caffeic acid 0.18 g; ferric citrate solution† 4.0 ml; agar 20.0 g; distilled H_2O 1000 ml. Autoclave at 121°C for 10 min.

MEDIA SUPPLEMENTS

These may be added to isolation media when contamination by bacteria or saprophytic fungi is likely to be troublesome. The antibacterial agent most commonly used is chloramphenicol at a concentration of 0.05 g/l. Cycloheximide (Actidione, Upjohn Co., Kalamazoo, Michigan) which inhibits the development of most common saprophytic fungi but does not inhibit a number of pathogens (e.g. dermatophytes) is also employed when necessary, at a concentration of 0.5 g/l.

* *Niger seed extract* obtained by pulverizing the seeds and adding 70 g seed powder to 350 ml distilled water. Autoclave at 121°C for 10 min and filter the aqueous extract through a gauze.

† *Ferric citrate solution.* Add 10.0 g ferric citrate to 20 ml distilled H_2O. Store in dark, discard if colour darkens.

They are the most conveniently added as follows:

50 mg chloramphenicol suspended in 10 ml 95% alcohol added to 1 l medium.

500 mg cycloheximide in 10 ml acetone added to 1 l medium.

Autoclave at 121°C for 10 min.

GLOSSARY

aleuriospore	terminal or lateral spore attached by a wide base and detached by fracture of the wall below the spore, e.g. microspores of dermatophytes
arthrospore	a spore resulting from the breaking up of a hypha into separate cells
ascocarp	a structure of varying complexity which bears sexual ascospores, found in the Ascomycotina
ascus	a sac-like cell in which sexual ascospores are produced
aseptate	lacking cross-walls
asexual	reproduction *not* involving union of two nuclei
asporogenous	non-spore forming
basidium	the structure, usually a single clavate cell, which after karyogamy and meiosis bears basidiospores
blastospore	a spore which has been budded off, as in the yeasts
chlamydospore	a thick-walled, intercalary or terminal cell containing stored food and able to function as a spore
cleistothecium	a sexual fruit-body (ascocarp) having no special opening
coenocytic	having many nuclei and few

	septa, as the hyphae of Phycomycetes
conidia	spores borne externally by fungi and which, when mature, detach from the conidiophore
coremium	a group of hyphae (or sporophores) generally upright and sometimes jointed together, producing spores
dematiaceous	hyphae and/or spores dark brown to black in colour
dimorphic	having two forms, as hyphal and yeast forms of certain pathogens
diploid	containing the double ($2n$) number of chromosomes
ectothrix	growth, usually in the form of a spore sheath on the surface of hair, as well as within the hair shaft
endospore	a spore borne within a cell, e.g. a sporangiospore
endothrix	growth within the hair shaft without a conspicuous external sheath of spores
gametangium	a structure which contains gametes
gamete	a sex cell
haploid	having the n or reduced number of chromosomes
heterothallic	a species in which 'sexes' are segregated and two different thalli are required for sexual reproduction
homothallic	species in which sexual reproduction takes place in a single thallus
hyaline	colourless, transparent
hypha	one of the filaments, septate or aseptate which go to make up the vegetative mycelium of fungi
macroconidium	the larger of two types of conidia in those fungi which produce large and small (microconidia) spores; it is usually multicellular
mycelium	the mass of hyphae making up the colony of a fungus
perfect state	the part of the life-cycle in which spores are formed after nuclear fusion (sexual reproduction)

peridium	the outside covering or wall of a fruiting body
phialide	a cell, usually more or less bottle shaped which forms conidia successively from its tip
pleomorphic	strictly having two or more forms; used frequently to describe a non-sporing (sterile) mutant in the dermatophytes
pseudophypha/ pseudomycelium	a fragile chain of cells (usually in yeasts), which have arisen by budding, with characteristics intermediate between a chain of yeast cells and a hypha
pseudoparenchyma	fungal tissue in which the component hyphae are not recognisable: cells are oval or isodiametric
pycnidium	fruit body, often flask-or bottle-shaped, within which are formed asexual conidia
sclerotium	a firm, frequently rounded mass of hyphae forming a resistant structure containing stored food
somatic	refers to the vegetative phase or structure as distinct from the reproductive
sporangium	a cell within which spores are borne by 'progressive cleavage'
sporophore	a spore-bearing structure
spore	a general name for a reproductive unit in cryptogams: in fungi frequently multicelled and may be sexual or asexual in origin
sterigma	a narrow pointed structure arising from a cell and supporting a spore
thallospore	an asexual spore produced directly, by septation of a hypha
thallus	the vegetative body
vesicle	a bladder-like sac: swollen portion of a hypha
zoospore	a motile asexually produced spore
zygospore	a resting spore which results from the fusion of two gametangia in the Zygomycotina
zygote	a diploid cell resulting from the union of two haploid cells

SELECTED BIBLIOGRAPHY

General mycology

Deacon J W 1980 Introduction to modern mycology. Blackwell Scientific, Oxford

Medical mycology

Chandler F W, Kaplan W, Ajello L 1980 Histopathology of mycotic diseases. A colour atlas and textbook. Wolfe Medical Atlases, London

Emmons C W, Binford C H, Utz J P, Kwon-Chung K J 1977 Medical mycology, 3rd edn. Lea and Febiger, Philadelphia

Odds F C 1979 Candida and candidosis. Leicester University Press, Leicester

Rippon J W 1982 Medical mycology. The pathogenic fungi and the pathogenic actinomyctes, 2nd edn. Saunders, Philadelphia

Speller D C E (ed) 1980 Antifungal chemotherapy. Wiley, Chichester

Stevens D A (ed) 1980 Coccidioidomycosis: A text. Plenum, New York

Warnock D W, Richardson M D (eds) 1982 Fungal infection in the compromised patient. Wiley, Chichester

Practical

Evans E G V (ed) 1976 Serology of fungal infection and Farmer's Lung disease. British Society for Mycopathology, University of Leeds Press

Mackenzie D W R, Philpot C M 1981 Isolation and identification of ringworm fungi. PHLS Monograph No. 15. HMSO, London

Mackenzie D W R, Philpot C M, Proctor A G J 1980 Basic serodiagnostic methods for diseases caused by fungi and actinomycetes. PHLS Monograph No. 12. HMSO, London

McGinnis M R 1980 Laboratory Handbook of Medical Mycology. Academic Press, New York

Palmer D F, Kaufman L, Kaplan W, Cavallaro J J 1977 Serodiagnosis of mycotic diseases. Charles C. Thomas, Springfield

INDEX